STAGE 4 BREAST CANCER DIET COOKBOOK

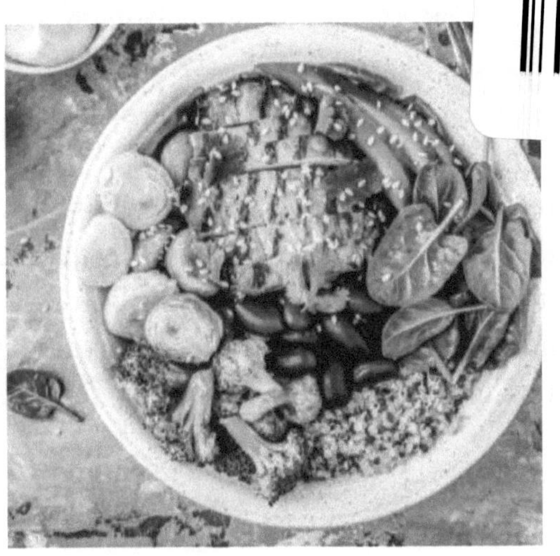

Discover the Benefits of Nourishing Your Body with Delicious Recipes Designed to Help Manage Stage 4 Breast Cancer and Improve Your Overall Health

Kathleen Scribner

Read more books by Kathleen Scribner by visiting:
https://www.amazon.com/author/skathleen234

The author has taken great care to present accurate and up-to-date information; however, the author and publisher do not assume any responsibility for errors or omissions or for the use or interpretation of the information contained herein.

TABLE OF CONTENTS

INTRODUCTION..5
Understanding Stage 4 Breast Cancer... 5
Importance of Nutrition in Cancer Treatment...........................10
CHAPTER ONE: PLANNING MEALS FOR OPTIMAL HEALTH.........17
Meal Planning Strategies..17
Portion Control and Eating Frequency......................................19
CHAPTER TWO: PRACTICAL TIPS FOR COOKING.............................23
Kitchen Tools and Gadgets for Easy Meal Preparation............. 23
Cooking Techniques to Retain Nutrients.................................... 26
CHAPTER THREE: SUPPORTING IMMUNE FUNCTION..29
Foods That Boost Immunity...29
Foods To Avoid.. 32
CHAPTER FOUR: DELICIOUS BREAKFAST RECIPES FOR MANAGING STAGE 4 BREAST CANCER............................. 36
CHAPTER FIVE: MOUTHWATERING LUNCH IDEAS FOR MANAGING STAGE 4 BREAST CANCER............................. 62
CHAPTER SIX: EASY AND DELICIOUS DINNER RECIPES FOR MANAGING STAGE 4 BREAST CANCER..................104
CHAPTER SEVEN: QUICK AND EASY SNACKS AND DESSERTS OPTION FOR MANAGING STAGE 4 BREAST CANCER...153
CHAPTER EIGHT: TASTY AND NUTRITIOUS SMOOTHIE RECIPES TO SOOTHE YOUR CRAVINGS......................171
CONCLUSION...186

INTRODUCTION

Understanding Stage 4 Breast Cancer

Stage 4 breast cancer, also known as metastatic breast cancer, is an advanced stage of breast cancer in which cancer cells have gone beyond the breast and surrounding lymph nodes to other areas of the body. This stage of cancer is distinguished by the occurrence of distant metastases, which often damage the bones, liver, lungs, or brain.

Causes and Risk Factors

The specific causes of breast cancer, especially its development to stage 4, are not well known. However, other risk factors have been found, including:

1. Genetic mutations: Inherited genetic mutations, such as those in the BRCA1 and BRCA2 genes, may raise the chance of developing breast cancer and impact its course.

2. Hormonal factors: Hormonal abnormalities, such as elevated levels of estrogen or progesterone, may contribute to the development and progression of breast cancer.

3. Lifestyle factors: Certain lifestyle choices, such as smoking, excessive alcohol use, a lack of physical exercise, and a poor diet, may raise the chance of developing breast cancer and progressing to stage 4.

4. Age and gender: Breast cancer is more frequent in women, especially those over the age of fifty. However, males may acquire breast cancer, albeit it is uncommon.

Symptoms

The symptoms of stage 4 breast cancer vary according to the location and amount of metastases. Common symptoms might include:

- Consistent breast lumps or changes in breast size or form.
- Swelling or soreness in the breasts or armpits, nipple discharge or inversion, and skin changes including redness, dimpling or thickness.
- Bone discomfort and fractures
- Shortness of breath or coughing, which indicates lung involvement.
- Abdominal discomfort or edema may indicate liver metastasis.
- Headaches, convulsions, or changes in mental state may indicate brain metastases.

It is essential to highlight that some people with stage 4 breast cancer may not have any symptoms at first, so early identification and continuous monitoring are critical for successful treatment.

Treatment Options

While stage 4 breast cancer is considered incurable, it may be controlled using a variety of therapeutic strategies targeted at symptom management, delaying disease progression, and enhancing quality of life. Treatment options might include:

1. Chemotherapy: Chemotherapy medications are used to destroy cancer cells and reduce tumors; they are often delivered in cycles or combinations.

2. Hormone therapy: Tamoxifen or aromatase inhibitors, which block hormones, may be used to treat hormone receptor-positive breast cancer.

3. Targeted therapy: Targeted medications, such as HER2-targeted treatments or CDK4/6 inhibitors, are intended to target cancer cells that have certain genetic alterations or features.

4. Radiation treatment: Radiation therapy may be used to alleviate pain or decrease tumors in regions impacted by metastases.

5. Surgery: In certain circumstances, surgery may be used to remove tumors or alleviate symptoms, such as bone metastases that cause fractures or spinal cord compression.

6. Palliative care: Palliative care aims to relieve symptoms and improve quality of life for people with advanced cancer, and it is often used in conjunction with other therapies.

Individuals with stage 4 breast cancer have a different prognosis dependent on variables such as the number of metastases, tumor features, therapy response, and general health. While stage 4 breast cancer is often incurable, advances in treatment choices have resulted in better survival rates and quality of life for many patients.

Understanding stage 4 breast cancer entails comprehending its intricacies, such as causes, symptoms, treatment choices, and prognosis. Individuals with stage 4 breast cancer may now get extensive assistance and individualized therapy to manage their illness and improve their well-being. Thanks to continuous research and medical improvements. We can continue to improve outcomes and quality of life for individuals impacted by this difficult condition by raising awareness, providing education, and increasing access to multidisciplinary treatment.

Importance of Nutrition in Cancer Treatment

Nutrition is essential in cancer therapy, especially for those with stage 4 breast cancer. Proper diet may aid with general health, treatment effectiveness, symptom management, and quality of life throughout the cancer journey. Here, we look at the significance of nutrition for people with stage 4 breast cancer, focusing on essential issues and solutions for appropriate nutritional support.

1. Supporting Overall Health: Proper nutrition is critical for overall health and well-being, particularly for people with stage 4 breast cancer, who may face issues such as tiredness, weight loss, and reduced immune function. A balanced diet rich in nutrient-dense foods delivers vital vitamins, minerals, antioxidants, and macronutrients required to support immune function, promote healing, and maintain strength and energy levels.

2. Improving Treatment Effectiveness: Nutrition is critical in maximizing the efficacy of cancer therapies such chemotherapy, hormone therapy, targeted therapy, and radiation therapy. Adequate diet helps the body to endure and recover from treatment-related adverse effects, reduces treatment delays and interruptions, and may enhance treatment results. For example, eating enough protein may assist sustain muscle building and tissue regeneration, while antioxidant-rich meals can help protect healthy cells from treatment-related harm.

3. Managing Symptoms: People with stage 4 breast cancer may have a variety of symptoms associated with both the disease and its treatment, such as nausea, vomiting, appetite loss, taste changes, mouth sores, constipation, diarrhea, and exhaustion. Proper eating may help reduce these symptoms and enhance overall quality of life. For example, eating small, frequent meals, keeping hydrated, avoiding hot or oily foods, and adding bland or calming alternatives may all assist with gastrointestinal issues. Working with a licensed dietitian or nutritionist may also result in individualized food suggestions to address particular symptoms and concerns.

4. Supporting Immune Function: Having a functional immune system is critical for people with stage 4 breast cancer because it helps the body fight against infections, promotes healing, and may slow cancer development. Nutrient-dense meals including fruits, vegetables, whole grains, lean meats, and healthy fats include vital vitamins, minerals, and antioxidants that help with immune function and general health. Furthermore, many dietary supplements, such as vitamin D, omega-3 fatty acids, and probiotics, may have immune-boosting properties when taken under the supervision of a healthcare expert.

5. Managing dietary Issues: People with stage 4 breast cancer may experience specific dietary issues that need specialist care and assistance. Appetite loss, taste alterations, trouble swallowing, gastrointestinal difficulties, weight loss, or unexpected weight gain are all possible concerns. Addressing these problems and developing a customized nutrition plan suited to individual requirements and preferences requires close collaboration with a multidisciplinary healthcare team that includes oncologists, registered dietitians, nurses, and other supportive care professionals.

6. Improving Quality of Life: Proper diet may dramatically improve the quality of life for people with stage 4 breast cancer by making them feel better physically, emotionally, and psychologically. Individuals who nourish their bodies with nutritious foods and address dietary concerns and challenges can experience increased energy levels, improved mood, better treatment tolerance, faster recovery from treatment-related side effects, and a greater sense of control and empowerment over their health and well-being.

Overcoming Stage 4 Breast Cancer Through Nutrition.

Despite the upheaval of her diagnosis, Jessica sought refuge in the quiet corners of her kitchen. Stage 4 breast cancer had thrown her into a maelstrom of uncertainty and anxiety, but behind those walls, she found a source of strength that would transform her life forever.

Jessica's journey started with a simple realization: food may be an ally in the battle against cancer. Armed with tenacity and a passion for information, she set out to discover the power of diet in treating her disease.
At first, the route seemed overwhelming. Jessica had several concerns and problems as she negotiated the minefield of contradicting information and fad diets. But

with effort and tenacity, she started to unearth the reality that lay behind the surface.

Jessica learnt via trial and error how to feed her body with meals that would help her battle cancer. **She adopted a diet rich in complete, nutrient-dense foods - vivid fruits and vegetables, lean meats, healthy fats, and fiber-rich grains - with each mouthful demonstrating her dedication to wellbeing.**

As the weeks passed into months, Jessica's efforts started to produce fruit. She felt stronger, more invigorated, more powerful than ever before. Her oncologist took note, marveling at her recovery and crediting much of it to her attention to food and nutrition.

But Jessica's alteration was more than simply physical; it affected every area of her existence. She delighted in the simple joys of cooking and sharing meals with loved ones. She gained a new sense of purpose by fighting for nutrition as an essential component of cancer treatment.

Jessica's spirit remained intact despite everything. She handled setbacks with elegance and fortitude, deriving courage from the fact that she was doing all she could to confront her sickness.

And then came a moment of triumph: Jessica's physician informed her that her tumor indicators had dramatically dropped. It was a success beyond her wildest expectations, demonstrating the transforming power of food and nutrition in her battle with stage 4 breast cancer.

Jessica is now a source of hope and inspiration for everyone who is going through similar struggles. Her tale serves as a reminder that even in the face of tragedy, there is always hope, and that everything is possible with the power of nutrition.

Through the pages of this cookbook, you can follow Jessica on her quest to overcome stage 4 breast cancer. Discover the tasty and healthy meals that kept her going, and let her tale inspire you to harness the transformational power of diet and nutrition in your own life.

In conclusion, the significance of nutrition in cancer therapy cannot be emphasized, especially for those dealing with stage 4 breast cancer. Individuals who prioritize healthy nutrition may promote general health, increase treatment efficacy, control symptoms, maintain immune function, address nutritional difficulties, and improve quality of life throughout their cancer journey, as Jessica did. Individuals may empower themselves to make educated food choices and enhance their nutritional well-being while navigating the difficulties of stage 4 breast cancer treatment and survival with information, advice, and individualized support.

CHAPTER ONE

PLANNING MEALS FOR OPTIMAL HEALTH

Meal Planning Strategies

Meal planning is a crucial part of treating Stage 4 breast cancer. A well-planned and healthy diet may help your body fight cancer while also managing treatment side effects. Here are some meal planning ideas that you may use to eat a balanced and healthy diet:

1. Plan Ahead: Set aside some time each week to plan your meals and snacks. This may help you remain on track with your nutritional objectives while also reducing the stress associated with mealtime selections. Try meal planning for the next week to ensure that you have healthy food alternatives accessible.

2. Focus on Nutrient-Dense Foods: Nutrient-dense foods are those that have a high concentration of important nutrients relative to their calorie level. Nutrient-dense foods include fruits and vegetables, entire grains, lean meats, and healthy fats. These meals may assist meet your body's nutritional requirements throughout cancer therapy.

3. Eat a Variety of meals: Eating a variety of meals guarantees that you are getting a wide range of critical nutrients. Incorporate items from all dietary categories into your meal plans, such as fruits, vegetables, whole grains, lean proteins, and healthy fats.

4. Consider Your Side Effects: Certain meals may aggravate cancer-related side effects such as nausea and vomiting. When preparing meals, keep your side effects in mind and go for items that are gentle on your stomach. For example, basic meals such as bread, crackers, and rice may aid with nausea.

5. Stay Hydrated: Staying hydrated is essential throughout cancer treatment. Aim for at least 8-10 glasses of water every day, and include hydrating items in your meals like melons and cucumbers.

6. Don't Forget About Snacks: Snacks may be an essential component of your meal planning approach. Healthy snack alternatives may help you stay satiated between meals while also providing energy. Consider snacks like fresh fruit, almonds, and yogurt.

7. Consult with a certified Dietitian: A certified dietitian may assist you in developing a personalized meal plan that takes into consideration your specific nutritional requirements and treatment plan. They may also provide advice and support during your treatment process.

8. Listen to Your Body: When planning and preparing meals, consider your body's indications and signals. Pay attention to hunger, fullness, and desires, and accept your body's demands and preferences without judgment. Eat consciously, relishing each mouthful, and consider how various meals affect you physically, emotionally, and cognitively.

Portion Control and Eating Frequency

Nutrition is critical in the management of stage 4 breast cancer because it improves general well-being and quality of life. As we negotiate the complexity of this path, it's critical to understand the fundamentals of portion control and eating frequency, as they are the foundation of a healthy and supporting diet.

Portion control is the technique of limiting the amount of food taken in each meal or snack. By paying attention to portion sizes, we may guarantee that our bodies get enough nutrients without overloading them with extra calories. For people with stage 4 breast cancer, portion management is even more important since maintaining a healthy weight and maximizing nutritional intake are top concerns.

One successful portion control method is to use visual clues and measurement equipment to determine optimal serving sizes. This might include using smaller plates and bowls to promote smaller servings, or measuring specified amounts of food using measuring cups or scales. Paying attention to hunger and fullness signals may also help reduce overeating and increase meal enjoyment.

Eating frequency, or the number of meals and snacks taken during the day, is just as essential as portion management. While there is no one-size-fits-all solution to eating frequency, evidence shows that dividing food consumption into smaller meals and snacks may help control blood sugar levels, boost energy, and reduce excessive hunger.

Incorporating regular, balanced meals and snacks into daily routines may offer a consistent supply of nutrition and fuel for those living with stage 4 breast cancer. Incorporate a variety of nutrient-dense meals at each meal, such as lean proteins, whole grains, fruits, vegetables, and healthy fats. This technique not only improves general health and nutrition, but also promotes energy stability and a feeling of well-being.

In addition to portion management and eating frequency, the quality of the meals ingested is a significant consideration. Incorporate whole, minimally processed foods into meals and snacks whenever feasible, while reducing your consumption of refined carbohydrates, saturated fats, and processed foods. By emphasizing nutrient-dense foods, we may give our bodies the vitamins, minerals, and antioxidants they need to boost immune function, maximize treatment results, and improve overall health.

As you begin your journey with the stage 4 breast cancer diet cookbook, I recommend approaching portion management and eating frequency with inquiry, awareness, and self-compassion. Listen to your body's cues, respect its particular demands, and remember that little, long-term improvements may reap substantial rewards.

May this serve as a guidepost as you negotiate the complexities of diet and wellbeing on your journey with stage 4 breast cancer. Let us all embrace portion restriction and eating frequency as useful tools for promoting health, vibrancy, and resilience.

CHAPTER TWO

PRACTICAL TIPS FOR COOKING

Kitchen Tools and Gadgets for Easy Meal Preparation

Meal preparation might be stressful at times when dealing with stage 4 breast cancer. However, having the proper kitchen equipment and gadgets may make the process much simpler and more pleasurable. Here's a list of crucial kitchen gear and devices that help make food preparation easier during this difficult time:

1. A high-quality blender or food processor is essential for making smoothies, soups, sauces, and purees. These multifunctional equipment can rapidly chop, combine, and puree items, making it easy to include nutrient-dense foods in your diet.

2. Instant Pot or Slow Cooker: Ideal for busy days or low energy levels. These gadgets let you create meals with little effort by just adding ingredients and cooking them gently over time.

3. Use sharp knives and cutting boards to safely and effectively chop, slice, and dice items. Investing in high-quality knives and cutting boards may make dinner preparation easier and more fun.

4. Vegetable Spiralizer: Incorporating more veggies into your meals is simple and enjoyable with a spiralizer. It lets you make noodles or ribbons from veggies such as zucchini, carrots, and sweet potatoes, which adds variety and nutrition to your meals.

5. Vegetable Steamer: A steamer is a useful tool for fast cooking vegetables while retaining their nutrition and taste. Simply pour water into the steamer, put the veggies in the basket, and steam until soft.

6. Salad Spinner: Use a salad spinner to easily wash and dry leafy greens. It helps to eliminate extra water from greens, keeping salads crisp and fresh.

7. Non-Stick Cookware: Non-stick cookware simplifies cooking and cleaning, particularly when energy is limited. Select high-quality, non-toxic cookware that is both durable and simple to use.

8. Measuring Cups and Spoons: Proper measuring is essential for effective cooking and baking. Keep a set of measuring cups and spoons on hand to guarantee accurate portion sizes and consistent outcomes.

9. Silicone Baking Mats and Muffin Liners: These non-stick, reusable mats and liners are eco-friendly and simple to clean. They're ideal for baking muffins, cookies, and other sweets without the need to grease pans or use disposable liners.

10. Kitchen Scale: Measuring by weight is more accurate than volume. It's especially useful for portion control and following recipes that need exact proportions.

These are just a handful of the necessary kitchen equipment and gadgets to make meal preparation simpler and more doable during the treatment of stage 4 breast cancer. By investing in these equipment and adopting them into your kitchen routine, you can simplify the cooking process, save time and energy, and concentrate on feeding your body with tasty and healthy meals.

Cooking Techniques to Retain Nutrients

As we begin the path of managing stage 4 breast cancer, fueling our bodies with nutrient-dense meals becomes critical. However, it is also critical to maintain the integrity of these nutrients throughout the cooking process. Here are several culinary strategies that may assist preserve the important nutrients need to sustain our health and well-being during this difficult time:

1. Steaming is a mild cooking technique that preserves the inherent tastes, colors, and nutrients of food. Steaming, which cooks vegetables and meats over simmering water, reduces nutritional loss compared to boiling or frying.

2. Sautéing and Stir-Fry: Sautéing and stir-frying cook dishes fast over high heat with a minimal quantity of oil. These methods retain the texture and nutritional value of foods while increasing the depth of flavor in recipes.

3. Baking and Roasting: Baking and roasting meals in the oven may improve taste and reduce nutritional loss. Roasting veggies, lean meats, and healthy grains at a moderate temperature preserves their vitamins, minerals, and antioxidants.

4. Grilling and Broiling: Cooking meals over an open flame or high heat source gives a smoky taste and caramelization without sacrificing nutrients. These approaches are ideal for lean proteins such as chicken, fish, and tofu.

5. Poaching: Foods are gently simmered in liquids like water, broth, or wine. This approach helps to maintain moisture and nutrients, making it suitable for delicate proteins such as fish and poultry.

6. Blend and puree fruits and vegetables to retain fiber and nutrients in smoothies, soups, and sauces. These strategies promote simple digestion and nutrition absorption, making them appropriate for those with poor digestive health.

7. Raw Preparation: Raw foods retain their inherent enzymes, vitamins, and minerals. Adding raw fruits, vegetables, nuts, and seeds to salads, snacks, and smoothies delivers a concentrated supply of nutrients and phytochemicals.

8. Minimal Processing: Chopping, slicing, or grating foods helps preserve their nutritious value. Avoiding excessive processing, such as peeling or juicing, protects the fiber and minerals inherent in whole foods.

By adopting these cooking methods into our culinary repertoire, we can increase the nutritional content of our meals while also providing our bodies with the vital elements required to promote our health and well-being throughout the treatment of stage 4 breast cancer.

CHAPTER THREE

SUPPORTING IMMUNE FUNCTION

Foods That Boost Immunity

When treating stage 4 breast cancer, it is critical to emphasize meals that promote immune function and general wellness. Here are some nutrient-rich meals that might help strengthen your immunity:

1. Colorful Fruits and Vegetables: Eat a range of colorful fruits and vegetables, including berries, citrus fruits, leafy greens, bell peppers, and sweet potatoes. These foods are high in vitamins, minerals, and antioxidants, which promote immune function and protect against inflammation.

2. Consume lean proteins including chicken, fish, tofu, beans, lentils, and Greek yogurt. Protein is required for the formation and repair of tissues, particularly those harmed by cancer therapy, and it also aids immunological function.

3. Consume healthy fats like avocados, nuts, seeds, and olive oil. These fats include omega-3 fatty acids and other nutrients that are anti-inflammatory and promote immunological health.

4. Choose whole grains, including brown rice, quinoa, oats, and whole wheat bread and pasta. Whole grains provide fiber, vitamins, and minerals, which promote general health and immunological function.

5. Incorporate probiotic-rich foods into your diet, including yogurt, kefir, sauerkraut, kimchi, and miso. Probiotics encourage the development of healthy gut bacteria, which aid in immunological control and digestion.

6. Garlic and onions contain sulfur compounds with antibacterial and immune-boosting qualities. Add them to soups, stews, stir-fries, and sauces to boost taste and immunity.

7. Ginger and Turmeric: Ginger and turmeric are recognized for their anti-inflammatory and antioxidant effects. Blend fresh ginger into smoothies, teas, and stir-fries, and add turmeric in curries, soups, and golden milk.

8. Mushrooms: Some mushrooms, including shiitake, maitake, and reishi, contain immune-modulating chemicals. Soups, stir-fries, omelets, and risottos are all great ways to use mushrooms.

9. Berries: Strawberries, blueberries, raspberries, and blackberries are high in antioxidants, vitamins, and fiber. Consume them fresh or frozen in smoothies, yogurt bowls, and salads.

10. Herbs and spices (e.g., parsley, cilantro, basil, oregano, cinnamon, and cayenne pepper) contain immune-boosting components. Use them freely while preparing and flavoring meals.

Including these nutrient-dense foods in your diet may assist boost immune function and general health throughout the treatment of stage 4 breast cancer. Remember to eat a well-balanced and varied diet, remain hydrated, and **get specialized nutritional guidance from a healthcare expert or certified dietitian.**

Foods To Avoid

When treating stage 4 breast cancer, it is essential to avoid certain foods that may have a detrimental impact on health or interfere with medications. Here are some items to restrict or avoid:

1. Processed and red meats: Processed meats, such as bacon, sausage, hot dogs, and deli meats, include chemicals and preservatives that may raise cancer risk. Red meats such as beef, hog, and lamb have significant levels of saturated fat, which may increase inflammation and contribute to cancer development.

2. Sugary Foods and Drinks: Sugary meals and drinks, including candy, pastries, sodas, and sweetened juices, may cause blood sugar rises and contribute to weight gain. Excess sugar intake has been related to inflammation, which may have a deleterious influence on cancer outcomes.

3. Highly processed foods: Fast food, packaged snacks, and frozen dinners are all examples of highly processed foods that include harmful fats, refined sugars, and added ingredients. These foods are deficient in vital nutrients and may lead to inflammation and chronic illnesses.

4. Fried and high-fat foods: Fried meals and foods rich in harmful fats, such as deep-fried snacks, fried chicken, and fatty cuts of meat, may cause inflammation and raise the risk of obesity and heart disease. Limiting your consumption of fried and high-fat meals is critical for general health.

5. Alcohol: Alcohol intake has been linked to an increased incidence of breast cancer and may have a detrimental influence on treatment results. Limiting or eliminating alcohol use may help lower cancer risk and improve general health.

6. Elevated-sodium meals including processed snacks, canned soups, and fast food may lead to elevated blood pressure and water retention. Excess salt consumption may potentially raise the risk of some malignancies and impair treatment success.

7. Artificial Sweeteners: Aspartame, saccharin, and sucralose are often used in diet drinks, sugar-free snacks, and processed meals. Some studies indicate that artificial sweeteners may have a deleterious impact on health and metabolism, although further study is required.

8. Trans Fats: Trans fats are present in partly hydrogenated oils used in processed and packaged meals. These fats may boost LDL (bad) cholesterol levels, increasing the risk of heart disease. Avoiding trans fat-containing meals is beneficial to general health.

9. Excessive Caffeine: While moderate caffeine use is usually regarded as safe, excessive consumption of caffeinated beverages such as coffee, tea, and energy drinks may lead to dehydration and disrupt sleep. Limiting caffeine use may improve general well-being.

10. Avoid eating unclean produce and raw seafood to lessen the risk of foodborne disease. This is particularly important for cancer patients with weaker immune systems.

Individuals dealing with stage 4 breast cancer may improve their overall health and well-being by avoiding certain foods and choosing better choices throughout treatment. For individualized nutritional recommendations suited to your specific requirements and preferences, **contact with a healthcare practitioner or registered dietitian.**

CHAPTER FOUR

DELICIOUS BREAKFAST RECIPES FOR MANAGING STAGE 4 BREAST CANCER

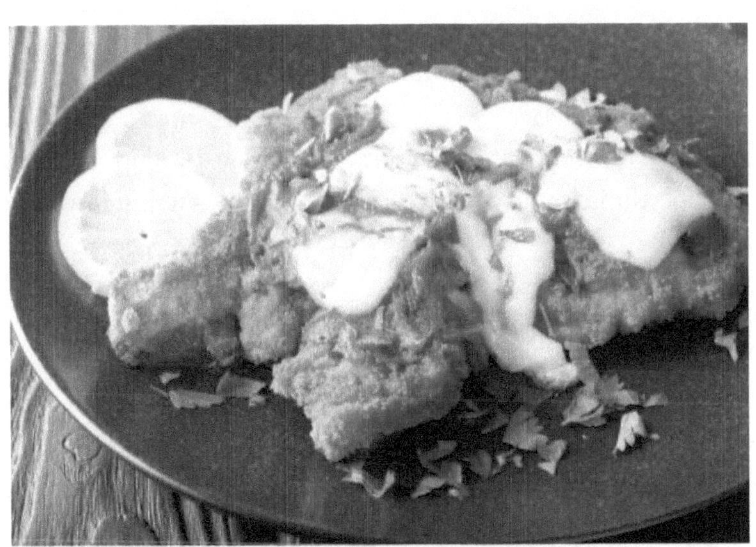

1. Oatmeal with Berries and Flax Seeds

Ingredients:

- 1 cup water
- 1/2 cup rolled oats
- 1/4 cup berries (fresh or frozen)
- 1 tablespoon ground flax seeds

Instructions:

1. Place one cup of water in a small pot and bring to a boil.
2. Lower the heat to medium and stir in 1/2 cup of rolled oats. Simmer for five to seven minutes, stirring now and again.
3. After cooking the oats, take them off the stove and mix it with 1/4 cup of frozen or fresh berries and 1 tablespoon of ground flaxseed.
4. Allow the berries to soften and release their juices by letting the oatmeal rest for a minute or two.
5. Garnish with flax seeds and berries, and savor your tasty and nourishing oatmeal!

2. Scrambled Eggs with Spinach and Whole Grain Toast

Ingredients:

- 2-3 eggs
- 1 handful of fresh spinach leaves
- 2 slices whole grain bread
- Salt and pepper to taste
- 1 tablespoon of butter or olive oil

Instructions:

1. Beat two to three eggs together in a small bowl with a dash of pepper and salt.
2. Turn on a medium heat source for a nonstick skillet. Add one tablespoon of either olive oil or butter to the pan.
3. After the butter or oil is hot, pour the egg mixture into the skillet after whisking. The eggs should be scrambled after being softly and evenly stirred with a spatula.
4. When the eggs are fully cooked and the spinach has wilted, add a handful of fresh spinach leaves to the skillet and stir the eggs occasionally.
5. Toast a couple of whole grain bread pieces.
6. Top the spinach-topped scrambled eggs with toasted whole grain bread and serve.

7. Savor your nutritious and delectable scrambled eggs with whole grain bread and spinach for breakfast!

3. Greek Yogurt with Nuts and Honey

Ingredients:

- 1 cup of Greek yogurt
- 1/4 cup of mixed nuts (almonds, walnuts, cashews, etc.)
- 1 tablespoon of honey

Instructions:

1. To begin, roast the nuts for three to five minutes over medium heat in a dry pan, or until they are aromatic and lightly browned. Allow it cool completely before chopping into tiny pieces.
2. The Greek yogurt should be scooped into a bowl.
3. Drizzle the yogurt with honey.
4. Top the yogurt and honey with a sprinkle of chopped nuts.
5. Using a spoon, combine all the ingredients.
6. Savor your nutritious and delectable Greek yogurt with honey and nuts!

4. Smoothie Bowl with Mixed Berries, Spinach, and Almond milk

Ingredients:

- 1 cup of mixed frozen berries (strawberries, raspberries, blueberries, etc.)
- 1 cup of fresh spinach leaves
- 1/2 cup of unsweetened almond milk
- 1 tablespoon of honey (optional)
- Toppings (granola, sliced fruit, chia seeds, etc.)

Instructions:

1. Place the fresh spinach leaves, almond milk, frozen mixed berries, and honey (if using) in a blender.
2. Use a high-speed blender to blend the ingredients until they are creamy and smooth. You may adjust the consistency by adding extra almond milk as required.
3. Transfer the smoothie blend into a bowl.
4. Top the smoothie with the preferred toppings (granola, sliced fruit, chia seeds, etc.).
5. Savor your nutritious and tasty smoothie bowl with spinach, almond milk, and mixed berries!

5. Avocado Toast with Smoked Salmon and Poached Egg

Ingredients:

- 2 slices of bread (whole wheat, sourdough, etc.)
- 1 ripe avocado
- 4 oz of smoked salmon
- 2 eggs
- 1 tablespoon of white vinegar
- Salt and pepper to taste

Instructions:

1. Toast the bread pieces until they are as crispy as you like.
2. Halve the avocado, remove the pit, and transfer the flesh to a bowl using a spoon.
3. Using a fork, mash the avocado and add salt and pepper to taste.
4. Evenly cover each piece of bread with mashed avocado.
5. Top the avocado spread with the smoked salmon, cut into tiny pieces.

6. Bring a saucepan of water to a simmer and add the white vinegar to poach the eggs.
7. Crack each egg into a ramekin or little dish.
8. Gently place each egg into the water that is simmering one at a time.
9. Cook the eggs for three to four minutes, or until the yolks are still runny but the whites are set.
10. Take the poached eggs out of the water using a slotted spoon.
11. Top each slice of bread with one poached egg.
12. To taste, add salt and pepper to the eggs.
13. Savor your nutritious and delectable avocado toast paired with poached eggs and smoked salmon!

6. Quinoa Bowl with Roasted Vegetables and a Soft Boiled Egg

Ingredients:

- 1 cup of cooked quinoa
- 2 cups of mixed vegetables (broccoli, bell peppers, zucchini, etc.), chopped
- 2 tablespoons of extra virgin olive oil
- Salt and pepper to taste
- 2 eggs

- Toppings (avocado slices, chopped nuts, etc.)

Instructions:

1. Set the oven's temperature to 400°F, or 200°C.
2. Arrange the diced veggies onto a baking sheet and lightly coat with extra virgin olive oil.
3. To taste, add salt and pepper to the veggies.
4. Bake the veggies for 20 to 25 minutes, or until they are soft and have a light brown hue.
5. Prepare the quinoa per the directions on the package while the veggies are roasting.
6. Bring a pot of water to a boil in order to soft boil the eggs.
7. Using a slotted spoon, carefully drop the eggs into the boiling water.
8. For a soft boiled egg, cook the eggs for six to seven minutes.
9. After taking the eggs out of the boiling water, give them a 30-second cooling soak in cold water.
10. Cut the eggs in half after peeling them.
11. Split the cooked quinoa into two bowls to make the quinoa bowl.
12. Arrange the roasted veggies on top of the quinoa.
13. Place the half-boiled soft eggs on top of the veggies.
14. Top the bowl with as many toppings as you like—sliced avocado, chopped nuts, etc.

15. Savor your nutritious and delectable quinoa meal topped with a soft-boiled egg and roasted veggies!

7. Whole Grain Waffles with Peanut Butter and Banana

Ingredients:

- 1 cup of whole wheat flour
- 2 tablespoons of brown sugar
- 2 teaspoons of baking powder
- 1/4 teaspoon of salt
- 1 cup of milk
- 1 egg
- 2 tablespoons of melted butter
- 1/2 teaspoon of vanilla extract
- Peanut butter
- Sliced bananas

Instructions:

1. Combine the whole wheat flour, baking powder, brown sugar, and salt in a mixing basin.
2. Combine the milk, egg, melted butter, and vanilla extract in another basin.

3. Combine the wet and dry ingredients, stirring just until blended.
4. Preheat a waffle iron and lightly grease with cooking spray.
5. Transfer the waffle batter into the waffle iron and cook it until golden brown and crispy, following the manufacturer's directions.
6. Place sliced bananas and a heaping dollop of peanut butter on top of the cooked waffles.
7. Present and savor your nutritious and delectable whole grain waffles with banana and peanut butter!

8. Vegetable Frittata with a Side of Fresh Fruit

Ingredients:

- 6 eggs
- 1/2 cup of milk
- 1/2 teaspoon of salt
- 1/4 teaspoon of black pepper
- 1 tablespoon of olive oil
- 1/2 cup of chopped onion
- 1 cup of mixed vegetables (spinach, bell peppers, mushrooms, etc.), chopped
- 1/2 cup of shredded cheese (cheddar, mozzarella, etc.)

- Fresh fruit (strawberries, blueberries, etc.) for serving

Instructions:

1. Set the oven's temperature to 175°C/350°F.
2. Combine the eggs, milk, salt, and black pepper in a mixing dish.
3. In a large ovenproof skillet, heat the olive oil over medium heat.
4. Cook the mixed veggies and chopped onion in the skillet for 5 to 7 minutes, or until the vegetables are soft.
5. Cover the veggies in the skillet with the egg mixture.
6. Scatter the cheese shreds on top of the egg mixture.
7. Place the skillet in the oven that has been warmed, and bake for 12 to 15 minutes, or until the cheese has melted and the eggs are set.
8. Take the skillet out of the oven and give it some time to cool.
9. Slice the frittata and serve it with a side of fresh fruit.
10. Savor your tasty and nutritious veggie frittata with a side of fresh fruit!

9. Chia Seed Pudding with Mixed Berries and Granola

Ingredients:

- 1/4 cup chia seeds
- 1 cup almond milk (or any milk of your choice)
- 1-2 tablespoons honey or maple syrup
- 1/2 teaspoon vanilla extract
- 1/2 cup mixed berries
- 1/4 cup granola

Instructions:

1. Combine the chia seeds, almond milk, vanilla extract, honey, or maple syrup, and mix them thoroughly in a medium-sized basin.
2. Refrigerate the bowl for a minimum of two hours or overnight, covered. After absorbing the liquid, the chia seeds will take on the consistency of pudding.
3. To serve, whisk the pudding and transfer it to a jar or serving dish.

Place mixed berries and granola on top. Additional toppings, such as chopped nuts or sliced bananas, are optional.

5. Put on a dish and savor!

10. Breakfast Burrito with Scrambled Eggs, Black Bean, and Salsa

Ingredients:

- 2 large eggs
- 1 tablespoon butter
- 1/4 cup black beans, drained and rinsed
- 2 tablespoons salsa
- 1 large flour tortilla

Instructions:

1. Beat the eggs well in a small basin.
2. Melt the butter in a nonstick pan over medium heat. Add the beaten eggs and heat until thoroughly cooked and scrambled, stirring from time to time.
3. Include the black beans in the skillet and stir to fully reheat.
4. Use a skillet or the microwave to reheat the tortilla.
5. In the center of the tortilla, put the black beans and scrambled eggs.
6. Place the salsa on top.
7. To construct a burrito, fold the tortilla's edges over the filling and roll it up from the bottom.
8. Present and savor!

11. Breakfast Wrap with Scrambled Eggs, Spinach, and Feta Cheese

Ingredients:

- 2 large eggs
- 1 tablespoon butter
- 1/2 cup fresh spinach leaves
- 1/4 cup crumbled feta cheese
- 1 large flour tortilla

Instructions:

1. Beat the eggs in a small bowl until thoroughly combined.
2. Melt the butter in a non-stick skillet over medium heat. After adding the beaten eggs, cook them, stirring now and then, until they are thoroughly cooked and scrambled.
3. Include the spinach leaves in the pan and toss to wilt them.
4. Use a skillet or microwave to reheat the tortilla.
5. In the center of the tortilla, place the spinach and scrambled eggs.
6. Garnish with feta cheese crumbles.

7. To create a wrap, fold the tortilla's edges over the filling and roll it up starting at the bottom.
8. Present and savor!

12. Protein Smoothie with Kale, Banana, and Almond Butter

Ingredients:

- 1 cup kale leaves, chopped
- 1 ripe banana, peeled and sliced
- 1 tablespoon almond butter
- 1 scoop vanilla protein powder
- 1 cup unsweetened almond milk (or any milk of your choice)
- 1/2 cup ice cubes

Instructions:

1. Fill a blender with the kale leaves, almond milk, protein powder, banana slices, and almond butter.
2. Blend on high for a smooth finish.
3. Blend one morc, adding the ice cubes, until smooth and creamy.
4. Immediately pour the smoothie into a glass and serve.

5. Savor the flavor and nutrition of your protein smoothie!

13. Overnight Oats with Mixed Berries and Almond Milk

Ingredients:

- 1/2 cup rolled oats
- 1/2 cup unsweetened almond milk (or any milk of your choice)
- 1/4 cup mixed berries
- 1 tablespoon honey or maple syrup (optional)
- 1/4 teaspoon vanilla extract (optional)

Instructions:

1. Place the rolled oats, almond milk, vanilla essence, honey, or maple syrup (if desired) in a small dish or container. Mix well to blend.
2. Gently swirl the mixed berries into the container to ensure that they are distributed evenly.
3. Put the jar in the fridge for the entire night (or for at least two hours) after covering it with a lid or plastic wrap.

4. Take the jar out of the fridge in the morning and mix the berries and oats. To thin down the mixture, add a small amount of almond milk if it's too thick.
5. Savor your wholesome and delectable overnight oats with almond milk and a variety of fruit!

14. Buckwheat Pancakes with Blueberries and Maple Syrup

Ingredients:

- 1 cup buckwheat flour
- 1/2 cup all-purpose flour
- 2 tablespoons sugar
- 2 teaspoons baking powder
- 1/2 teaspoon salt
- 1 1/2 cups milk
- 2 eggs
- 2 tablespoons vegetable oil
- 1 cup fresh blueberries
- Maple syrup, for serving

Instructions:

1. Combine the buckwheat flour, all-purpose flour, sugar, baking powder, and salt in a large basin.

2. Whisk the eggs, milk, and vegetable oil in another bowl.
3. Combine the wet and dry ingredients, stirring just until blended. Take caution not to blend too much.
4. Fold the blueberries in gently.
5. Turn up the heat to medium on a nonstick skillet or griddle.
6. Transfer the batter on the pan or griddle using a 1/4 cup measuring.
7. Cook the pancake until bubbles appear on the surface and the edges start to dry. Then, turn it over and continue cooking until the second side is golden brown.
8. Continue with the leftover batter.
9. Drizzle some maple syrup over the warm pancakes. Enjoy!

15. Poached Eggs on Whole Grain Toast with Sliced Avocado

Ingredients:

- 2 large eggs
- 2 slices of whole grain bread
- 1 avocado, sliced
- Salt and pepper to taste
- Vinegar (optional)

Instructions:

1. Toast the bread slices until they are golden brown and crispy.
2. While the bread is toasting, bring a pot of water to a simmer.
3. Add a splash of vinegar to the water (optional). The vinegar helps the egg whites to set more quickly and prevents them from spreading.
4. Crack the eggs into two separate cups.
5. Use a spoon to create a whirlpool in the simmering water.
6. Gently pour one egg into the center of the whirlpool. Repeat with the other egg.
7. Cook the eggs until the yolks are still runny and the whites are set, about 3 to 4 minutes.
8. To drain any extra water, take the eggs out of the water using a slotted spoon and set them on a paper towel.
9. Transfer the slices of toast to a platter.
10. Add avocado slices to the top of each slice.
11. On top of every slice of bread, place a poached egg.
12. Top the eggs with a little salt and pepper.
13. Savor your healthy and tasty breakfast!

16. Cottage Cheese with Sliced Peaches and a Sprinkle of Cinnamon

Ingredients:

- 1/2 cup cottage cheese
- 1 ripe peach, sliced
- A sprinkle of ground cinnamon

Instructions:

1. Fill a dish with the cottage cheese.
2. Clean the peach and cut it into thin slices.
3. Place the pieces of peach over the cottage cheese.
4. Garnish the top with a small sprinkle of ground cinnamon.
5. Savor your tasty and nutritious breakfast!

17. Breakfast Bowl with Quinoa, Roasted Sweet Potatoes, and a Fried egg

Ingredients:

- 1/2 cup quinoa
- 1 medium sweet potato, cubed
- 1 tablespoon olive oil
- Salt and pepper to taste
- 1 large egg
- **Optional toppings:** sliced avocado, chopped green onions, hot sauce

Instructions:

1. Turn the oven on to 400°F, or 200°C.
2. Place the rinsed quinoa in a colander with fine mesh and add one cup of water to the saucepan. Once the water is absorbed and the quinoa is soft, bring to a boil, then lower the heat to a simmer for 15 to 20 minutes.
3. Toss the diced sweet potato with salt, pepper, and olive oil while the quinoa cooks. Arrange the sweet potatoes on a baking sheet in a single layer, then bake for 20 to 25 minutes, or until they become soft and start to turn a light shade of brown.
4. Fry one egg to the doneness you desire in a non-stick skillet.
5. To make the breakfast bowl, transfer the roasted sweet potatoes and cooked quinoa to a bowl.
6. Add the fried egg on top.
7. You may also add other toppings like spicy sauce, chopped green onions, or sliced avocado.
8. Savor your wholesome and filling breakfast bowl!

18. Veggie Omelet with Mushrooms, Onions, and Peppers

Ingredients:

- 2 large eggs
- 1/4 cup chopped mushrooms
- 1/4 cup chopped onions
- 1/4 cup chopped bell peppers
- 1 tablespoon olive oil
- Salt and pepper to taste
- **Optional toppings:** shredded cheese, chopped fresh herbs

Instructions:

1. Beat the eggs with a fork in a small bowl until thoroughly combined. Add pepper and salt according to taste.
2. In a nonstick skillet set over medium-high heat, warm the olive oil.
3. Add the chopped bell peppers, onions, and mushrooms to the skillet and sauté for three to four minutes, or until the veggies are soft.

4. To distribute the eggs equally, pour the beaten eggs into the skillet and tilt the pan.
5. Until the edges begin to set, cook the eggs without stirring for one to two minutes.
6. To allow the raw eggs to flow to the pan's edges, raise the omelet's edges with a spatula.
7. Fold the omelet in half using the spatula when the eggs are almost done but still a little runny on top.
8. Cook the eggs for a further one to two minutes, or until they are cooked to your desired consistency.
9. Transfer the omelet to a platter and, if like, top with chopped fresh herbs and grated cheese.
10. Plate hot and savor your tasty vegetarian omelet!

19. Whole Grain Bagel with Cream Cheese and Smoked Salmon

Ingredients:

- 1 whole grain bagel, sliced in half
- 2 ounces smoked salmon
- 2 tablespoons cream cheese
- Sliced red onion (optional)
- Capers (optional)

Instructions:

1. Toast the slices of whole grain bagel until they get crispy and golden brown.
2. Top each half of a bagel with a thick coating of cream cheese.
3. Place a couple slices of smoked salmon on top of each slice.
4. You may garnish with a few red onion slices and a sprinkling of capers, if you'd like.
5. Present and savor your scrumptious and nutritious brunch or breakfast!

20. Homemade Granola with Greek Yogurt and Fresh Fruit

Ingredients for Homemade Granola:

- 2 cups old-fashioned rolled oats
- 1/2 cup chopped nuts (such as almonds, pecans, or walnuts)
- 1/2 cup unsweetened shredded coconut
- 1/4 cup honey
- 1/4 cup coconut oil, melted
- 1 teaspoon vanilla extract
- 1/2 teaspoon ground cinnamon

- Pinch of salt

Ingredients for Serving:

- 1/2 cup Greek yogurt
- 1/2 cup fresh fruit (such as berries, sliced bananas, or chopped apples)

Instructions for Homemade Granola:

1. Set the oven's temperature to 150°C/300°F.
2. Combine the rolled oats, chopped nuts, shredded coconut, ground cinnamon, and salt in a large bowl.
3. Combine the honey, melted coconut oil, and vanilla extract in another bowl.
4. Once the oat mixture is fully cooked, pour the honey mixture over it and stir.
5. On a baking sheet covered with parchment paper, distribute the granola mixture in a uniform layer.
6. Bake the granola for 20 to 25 minutes, stirring now and again, until it becomes crispy and golden brown.
7. Before serving or storing, let the granola cool fully on the baking pan.

Instructions for Serving:

1. Transfer the Greek yogurt into a bowl using a spoon.

2. Scatter a heaping portion of the homemade granola over the yogurt.
3. Place some fresh fruit on top of the granola.
4. Present your delectable and nutritious breakfast and savor it!

CHAPTER FIVE

MOUTHWATERING LUNCH IDEAS FOR MANAGING STAGE 4 BREAST CANCER

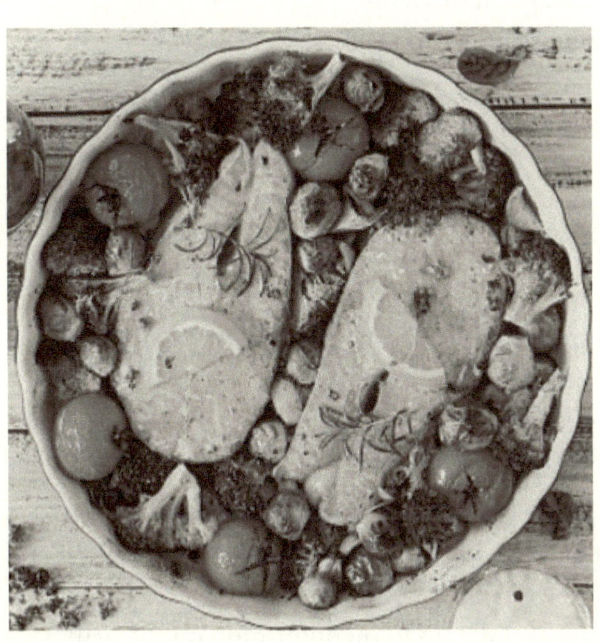

1. Grilled Chicken and Vegetable Skewers with Quinoa Salad

Ingredients for Chicken and Vegetable Skewers:

- 2 boneless, skinless chicken breasts, cut into cubes
- 1 red bell pepper, cut into chunks
- 1 yellow bell pepper, cut into chunks
- 1 red onion, cut into chunks
- 8-10 wooden skewers, soaked in water for 30 minutes
- 1 tablespoon olive oil
- Salt and pepper to taste

Ingredients for Quinoa Salad:

- 1 cup cooked quinoa
- 1/2 cup diced cucumber
- 1/2 cup cherry tomatoes, halved
- 1/4 cup chopped fresh parsley
- 2 tablespoons lemon juice
- 2 tablespoons olive oil
- Salt and pepper to taste

Instructions for Chicken and Vegetable Skewers:

1. Turn the heat up to medium-high on the grill.

2. Alternately thread the bell peppers, onions, and chicken onto the skewers.
3. Add salt and pepper to the skewers after brushing them with olive oil.
4. Cook, rotating the skewers every 12 to 15 minutes, or until the veggies are soft and well browned and the chicken is cooked through.
5. Before serving, take the skewers off the grill and allow them to cool for a few minutes.

Instructions for Quinoa Salad:

1. Put the cooked quinoa, diced cucumber, cut cherry tomatoes in half, and chopped fresh parsley in a big bowl.
2. Combine the lemon juice, olive oil, salt, and pepper in a small bowl.
3. Drizzle the quinoa salad with the dressing and mix thoroughly.
4. Present the quinoa salad beside the chicken and veggie skewers.
5. Savor your tasty and nutritious lunch!

2. Lentil Soup with a Side of Mixed Green Salad

Ingredients for Lentil Soup:

- 1 cup dried brown lentils, rinsed and drained
- 1 tablespoon olive oil
- 1 onion, chopped
- 3 garlic cloves, minced
- 1 carrot, peeled and chopped
- 1 celery stalk, chopped
- 4 cups vegetable broth or chicken broth
- 1 bay leaf
- 1 teaspoon ground cumin
- 1/2 teaspoon ground coriander
- Salt and pepper to taste
- Fresh lemon juice (optional)

Ingredients for Mixed Green Salad:

- 4 cups mixed greens (such as lettuce, spinach, and arugula)
- 1/2 cup cherry tomatoes, halved
- 1/2 cup chopped cucumber
- 2 tablespoons balsamic vinaigrette

Instructions for Lentil Soup:

1. Heat the olive oil in a big saucepan over medium heat.

2. Add the minced garlic and chopped onion, and sauté for two to three minutes, or until the onion becomes transparent.
3. Sauté the chopped celery and carrot for a further two to three minutes.
4. Fill the saucepan with the washed and drained lentils, stirring to mix.
5. Fill the saucepan with the vegetable or chicken broth, bay leaf, ground coriander, ground cumin, and salt and pepper, and stir to mix.
6. After bringing the soup to a boil, lower the heat to a simmer and cook for 30 to 35 minutes, or until the lentils are soft and the flavors have combined.
7. Take out the bay leaf from the soup and adjust the seasoning by adding more salt, pepper, and, if desired, fresh lemon juice to taste.

Instructions for Mixed Green Salad:

1. Put the diced cucumber, halved cherry tomatoes, and mixed greens in a big bowl.
2. Cover the salad with the balsamic vinaigrette and toss to mix.

To Serve:

1. Spoon the hot lentil soup into individual bowls.
2. Present the mixed green salad as an accompaniment.

3. Savor your tasty and nutritious lunch!

3. Salmon Salad Wraps with Whole Grain Tortillas

Ingredients for Salmon Salad:

- 2 cooked salmon filets, flaked
- 1/4 cup plain Greek yogurt
- 1 tablespoon mayonnaise
- 1 tablespoon Dijon mustard
- 1 tablespoon lemon juice
- 1/4 cup chopped celery
- 1/4 cup chopped red onion
- Salt and pepper to taste

Ingredients for Wraps:

- 4 whole grain tortillas
- 1 cup mixed greens
- 1/2 cup sliced cucumber
- 1/2 cup sliced avocado

Instructions for Salmon Salad:

1. Combine the Greek yogurt, lemon juice, Dijon mustard, and mayonnaise in a medium-sized bowl.
2. Transfer the chopped celery and red onion to the bowl along with the cooked and flaked salmon, and mix everything together.
3. To taste, add salt and pepper to the salmon salad.

Instructions for Wraps:

1. On a level surface, arrange the whole grain tortillas.
2. Evenly distribute the salmon salad among the tortillas, arranging it in a central row.
3. Place a few sliced avocado, cucumber, and mixed greens on top of each tortilla.
4. Tuck the sides in as you carefully roll up the tortillas.
5. Cut the wraps in half on the diagonal before serving.

4. Turkey and Avocado Sandwiches on Whole Wheat Bread

Ingredients:

- Sliced turkey breast (cooked or deli-style)
- Ripe avocado, thinly sliced or mashed
- Whole wheat bread slices

- Lettuce leaves
- Tomato slices
- **Optional:** sliced red onion, mustard, mayonnaise, cheese slices

Instructions:

1. If preferred, start by toasting the pieces of whole wheat bread.
2. Top each piece of bread with a layer of mashed avocado. As an alternative, you may just put the thinly sliced avocado right on the toast.
3. Evenly top the avocado with a layer of sliced turkey breast on one side of the bread.
4. Place tomato slices and lettuce leaves over the turkey.
5. You may optionally add extras like cheese slices, mayonnaise, mustard, and chopped red onion.
6. To assemble sandwiches, place the remaining bread slices on top.
7. To make handling the sandwiches simpler, you can choose to cut them in half horizontally or diagonally.
8. Present the turkey and avocado sandwiches right away, and experience the combination of crunchy veggies, flavorful turkey, and creamy avocado sandwiched between thick pieces of good wheat bread.

5. Roasted vegetable and chickpea Buddha bowls

Ingredients:

For the Roasted Vegetables:

- 2 cups mixed vegetables (such as bell peppers, zucchini, carrots, broccoli, cauliflower), chopped
- 1 can chickpeas, drained and rinsed
- 2 tablespoons olive oil
- 1 teaspoon garlic powder
- 1 teaspoon dried herbs (such as thyme, rosemary, or oregano)
- Salt and pepper to taste

For the Quinoa:

- 1 cup quinoa, rinsed
- 2 cups water or vegetable broth
- Salt to taste

For the Avocado Dressing:

- 1 ripe avocado
- Juice of 1 lime
- 2 tablespoons olive oil

- 1 clove garlic, minced
- 1/4 cup fresh cilantro, chopped
- Salt and pepper to taste
- Water, as needed to thin the dressing

Optional Toppings:

- Sliced avocado
- Cherry tomatoes, halved
- Sliced radishes
- Sprouts or microgreens
- Toasted seeds or nuts (such as pumpkin seeds or almonds)
- Crumbled feta cheese

Instructions:

1. Set the oven temperature to 400°F, or 200°C. Use silicone baking mats or parchment paper to line a baking pan.
2. Add the chopped mixed veggies and chickpeas to a large mixing bowl and toss to cover evenly with the olive oil, dry herbs, garlic powder, salt, and pepper.
3. Evenly distribute the vegetable and chickpea mixture onto the baking sheet that has been prepared.
4. Roast, stirring halfway through, in the preheated oven for 25 to 30 minutes, or until the veggies are soft and gently browned.

5. Make the quinoa while the veggies are roasting. Rinse the quinoa and put it in a medium pot with either water or vegetable broth. After bringing to a boil, lower the heat to a simmer, cover, and cook the quinoa for 15 to 20 minutes, or until it is tender and the liquid has been absorbed. Using a fork, fluff the mixture and add salt to taste.
6. In a blender or food processor, blend the avocado flesh, lime juice, olive oil, minced garlic, chopped cilantro, salt, and pepper to make the avocado dressing. Add water as necessary to get the required consistency and blend until smooth.
7. Distribute the cooked quinoa among serving dishes to assemble the Buddha bowls. Place the combination of roasted vegetables and chickpeas on top.
8. Spoon the avocado dressing over each bowl or pass it separately.
9. Optional garnishes for the bowls are chopped feta cheese, sprouts or microgreens, cherry tomatoes, sliced radishes, sliced avocado, and toasted seeds or almonds.
10. Present the Buddha bowls with roasted vegetables and chickpeas right away, then savor the delectable tastes and textures of this filling dish.

6. Tuna Salad Stuffed Bell Peppers

Ingredients:

- 4 large bell peppers (any color), halved and seeds removed
- 2 cans (5 oz each) tuna, drained
- 1/2 cup plain Greek yogurt or mayonnaise
- 1 tablespoon Dijon mustard
- 1/4 cup red onion, finely chopped
- 1/4 cup celery, finely chopped
- 1/4 cup cucumber, finely chopped
- 1/4 cup carrot, grated
- 2 tablespoons fresh parsley, chopped
- Juice of 1 lemon
- Salt and pepper to taste
- **Optional toppings:** sliced cherry tomatoes, avocado slices, olives, feta cheese, chopped herbs

Instructions:

1. Set the oven temperature to 375°F, or 190°C. Grease a baking dish gently with olive oil or line it with parchment paper.
2. Put the bell pepper halves, cut side up, in the baking dish that has been prepared.
3. Place the drained tuna, Greek yogurt or mayonnaise, Dijon mustard, chopped celery, cucumber, red onion,

grated carrot, chopped parsley, lemon juice, salt, and pepper in a big mixing bowl. Mix until well blended.

4. Evenly spoon the tuna salad mixture into each half of a bell pepper, gently pushing to fill; do not press down too much.
5. Cover the baking dish with aluminum foil, and bake the dish in the preheated oven for 20 to 25 minutes, or until the mixture is well cooked and the bell peppers are soft.
6. Take off the foil and bake for a further five to ten minutes, or until the tops start to turn a light shade of golden brown.
7. When the filled bell peppers are done, take them out of the oven and allow them to cool a little before serving.
8. Add optional toppings to the tuna salad-stuffed bell peppers, including chopped herbs, avocado slices, olives, and sliced cherry tomatoes.
9. Enjoy the delectable mix of soft bell peppers and savory tuna salad filling as you serve the stuffed bell peppers warm or at room temperature.

7. Veggie Stir-Fry with Tofu and Brown Rice

Ingredients:

For the Stir-Fry:

- 1 block (14 oz) firm tofu, pressed and cubed
- 2 tablespoons soy sauce or tamari
- 1 tablespoon sesame oil
- 2 tablespoons olive oil or vegetable oil
- 2 cloves garlic, minced
- 1 tablespoon ginger, minced
- 1 onion, sliced
- 2 bell peppers, sliced (any color)
- 2 carrots, julienned
- 1 cup broccoli florets
- 1 cup snap peas or snow peas
- 1 cup mushrooms, sliced
- Salt and pepper to taste

For the Sauce:

- 1/4 cup low-sodium soy sauce or tamari
- 2 tablespoons rice vinegar
- 1 tablespoon honey or maple syrup
- 1 teaspoon sesame oil
- 1 teaspoon cornstarch
- **Optional:** red pepper flakes for heat

For Serving:

- Cooked brown rice

- **Optional garnishes:** sliced green onions, sesame seeds, cilantro

Instructions:

1. Begin by pressing the blocked tofu between two clean kitchen towels or paper towels. To remove excess moisture, set a heavy item, such as a stack of plates or a cast-iron pan, on top of the tofu and leave for 15 to 30 minutes. Press the tofu and chop it into pieces.
2. In a small bowl, combine the sesame oil and soy sauce/tamari. After evenly coating the tofu cubes, put them in the marinade and let them sit for ten to fifteen minutes.
3. In the meanwhile, combine the cornstarch, sesame oil, rice vinegar, honey or maple syrup, and soy sauce or tamari in a small dish. Put aside.
4. In a large skillet or wok, heat one tablespoon of vegetable or olive oil over medium-high. Add the marinated tofu cubes and cook for 5 to 7 minutes, or until golden brown and crisp on both sides. After removing the tofu from the pan, put it aside.
5. If required, add an additional tablespoon of oil to the same skillet. Sauté the ginger and garlic for one to two minutes, until fragrant.
6. In the pan, combine the bell peppers, carrots, broccoli florets, snap peas, onion slices, and mushrooms. Stir-fry

the vegetables for five to seven minutes, or until crisp tender.

7. Return the cooked tofu and vegetables to the skillet. After pouring the sauce over the tofu and vegetables, swirl to ensure that they are evenly covered. Simmer for another two to three minutes, or until the sauce is somewhat thickened.

8. Season the stir-fry to taste with salt, pepper, and optional red pepper flakes.

9. Serve the warm veggie stir-fry over cooked brown rice. If desired, sprinkle with cilantro, sesame seeds, and sliced green onions.

10. Serve this delectable and nutritious stir-fried vegetable meal with brown rice and tofu for a satisfying lunch or supper.

8. Spinach and Feta Stuffed Chicken Breasts with Roasted Sweet Potatoes

Ingredients:

For the Spinach and Feta Stuffed Chicken Breasts:

- 4 boneless, skinless chicken breasts
- 2 cups fresh spinach leaves, chopped

- 1/2 cup crumbled feta cheese
- 2 cloves garlic, minced
- 1 tablespoon olive oil
- Salt and pepper to taste

For the Roasted Sweet Potatoes:

- 2 large sweet potatoes, peeled and cubed
- 2 tablespoons olive oil
- 1 teaspoon paprika
- 1 teaspoon garlic powder
- Salt and pepper to taste

Instructions:

1. Set the oven temperature to 375°F, or 190°C. Use aluminum foil or parchment paper to line a baking pan.
2. Get the stuffing of spinach and feta ready: One tablespoon of olive oil should be heated over medium heat in a skillet. Add the chopped spinach and minced garlic; sauté for 2 to 3 minutes, or until the spinach wilts. Take off the heat and let it cool a little.
3. Place the crumbled feta cheese and the sautéed spinach mixture in a mixing bowl. To taste, add salt and pepper for seasoning.
4. To create a pocket for the stuffing, cut a horizontal slit down the side of each chicken breast with a sharp knife.

5. Divide the spinach and feta mixture equally among the chicken breasts and stuff each one. If necessary, use toothpicks to seal the holes.
6. Transfer the filled chicken breasts to the baking sheet that has been ready.
7. Combine the cubed sweet potatoes, olive oil, paprika, garlic powder, salt, and pepper in a separate mixing basin and toss until well coated.
8. Arrange the seasoned sweet potatoes around the chicken breasts on the baking pan in a single layer.
9. Roast, turning the sweet potatoes midway through, in a preheated oven for 25 to 30 minutes, or until the chicken is cooked through and they are soft.
10. Take the roasted sweet potatoes and filled chicken breasts out of the oven once they are done.
11. Before serving, let the chicken rest for a few minutes. Before serving, take the toothpicks out.
12. Present the feta and spinach-stuffed chicken breasts with the roasted sweet potatoes on the side.
13. Savor this tasty and nutritious meal that includes flawlessly roasted sweet potatoes and soft chicken breasts packed with savory spinach and feta.

9. Caprese Salad with Grilled Chicken

Ingredients:

For the grilled chicken:

- 4 boneless, skinless chicken breasts
- 2 tablespoons olive oil
- 2 cloves garlic, minced
- 1 teaspoon dried Italian herbs (such as basil, oregano, thyme)
- Salt and pepper to taste

For the Caprese salad:

- 2 large ripe tomatoes, sliced
- 1 ball fresh mozzarella cheese, sliced
- Fresh basil leaves
- Balsamic glaze or reduction
- Salt and pepper to taste

Instructions:

1. Turn the heat up to medium-high on your grill.
2. To make a marinade for the chicken, combine the olive oil, minced garlic, dried Italian herbs, salt, and pepper in a small bowl.
3. Put the chicken breasts in a plastic bag that can be sealed or in a shallow plate. Make sure that every breast of chicken is equally covered when you pour the

marinade over it. For optimal taste, marinate for at least 30 minutes or up to 4 hours in the refrigerator.

4. Prepare the ingredients for the caprese salad while the chicken marinades. Cut the fresh mozzarella cheese and tomatoes into rounds of the same size. On a serving dish, arrange the tomato and mozzarella slices in alternating rows, slightly overlapped. Place a few fresh basil leaves in between the cheese and tomato pieces.

5. Add salt and pepper to taste and drizzle the caprese salad with a balsamic glaze or reduction. Store until you're ready to serve.

6. Take the chicken out of the marinade when it has completed marinating, discarding any extra marinade.

7. Cook the chicken breasts for 6 to 8 minutes on each side, or until they are cooked through and no longer have a pink center, over a preheated grill. The chicken should be cooked through to an internal temperature of 165°F (74°C).

8. Before slicing, take the grilled chicken from the grill and let it sit for a few minutes.

9. Top the prepared Caprese salad with the sliced grilled chicken to serve.

10. If wanted, garnish with more fresh basil leaves and a balsamic glaze drizzle.

11. Savor this mouthwatering and filling Caprese salad with grilled chicken, which has savory grilled chicken, creamy mozzarella, and juicy tomatoes.

10. Mediterranean Quinoa Salad with Grilled Shrimp

Ingredients:

- 1 cup quinoa, cooked and cooled
- 1 pound large shrimp, peeled and deveined
- 1 cup cherry tomatoes, halved
- 1 cucumber, diced
- 1/2 red onion, finely chopped
- 1/4 cup Kalamata olives, sliced
- 1/4 cup feta cheese, crumbled
- 1/4 cup fresh parsley, chopped
- 3 tablespoons extra virgin olive oil
- 2 tablespoons red wine vinegar
- 1 teaspoon dried oregano
- Salt and pepper to taste
- Lemon wedges for serving

Instructions:

1. Turn the heat up to medium-high on the grill or grill pan.
2. Combine shrimp, salt, and pepper in a bowl and mix. Drizzle with olive oil.

3. Grill shrimp for two to three minutes on each side, or until they are cooked through and have a hint of sear.
4. Put the cooked quinoa, cherry tomatoes, cucumber, red onion, feta, olives, and parsley in a big mixing dish.
5. Combine the olive oil, red wine vinegar, salt, pepper, and dried oregano in a small dish.
6. Drizzle the quinoa mixture with the dressing and stir thoroughly.
7. Add grilled shrimp to the top of the quinoa salad.
8. Present the Mediterranean Quinoa Salad accompanied by wedges of lemon.

11. Black Bean and Corn Salad with Grilled Fish

Ingredients:

For the Salad:

- 1 can (15 oz) black beans, drained and rinsed
- 1 cup corn kernels (fresh or thawed if using frozen)
- 1 red bell pepper, diced
- 1/2 red onion, finely chopped
- 1 cup cherry tomatoes, halved
- 1/4 cup fresh cilantro, chopped

For the Grilled Fish:

- 4 fish filets (such as tilapia, mahi-mahi, or cod)
- 2 tablespoons olive oil
- 1 teaspoon ground cumin
- 1 teaspoon paprika
- Salt and pepper to taste
- Lime wedges for serving

For the Lime Vinaigrette:

- 3 tablespoons olive oil
- 2 tablespoons fresh lime juice
- 1 teaspoon honey or agave syrup
- Salt and pepper to taste

Instructions:

1. Turn the heat up to medium-high on the grill or grill pan.
2. Put the black beans, corn, cherry tomatoes, red bell pepper, red onion, and cilantro in a big bowl.
3. Combine the olive oil, paprika, ground cumin, salt, and pepper in a small bowl. Use this mixture to lightly coat the fish filets.
4. Cook the fish filets on the grill for 3–4 minutes on each side, or until they are cooked through and have grill marks.

5. In the meantime, mix olive oil, lime juice, honey (or agave syrup), salt, and pepper to make the lime vinaigrette.
6. Break the fish into little pieces when it's done.
7. Top the black bean and corn salad with the grilled fish. After adding the lime vinaigrette to the salad, gently toss to mix.
8. Present the grilled fish with the black bean and corn salad right away, and top with lime wedges.

12. Turkey Meatball and Vegetables Soup

Ingredients:

For the Turkey Meatballs:

- 1 pound ground turkey
- 1/2 cup breadcrumbs
- 1/4 cup grated Parmesan cheese
- 1 large egg
- 2 cloves garlic, minced
- 1 teaspoon dried oregano
- Salt and pepper to taste

For the Soup:

- 1 tablespoon olive oil
- 1 onion, diced
- 2 carrots, sliced
- 2 celery stalks, sliced
- 3 cloves garlic, minced
- 1 zucchini, diced
- 1 can (14 oz) diced tomatoes
- 6 cups low-sodium chicken broth
- 1 teaspoon dried thyme
- 1 teaspoon dried rosemary
- Salt and pepper to taste
- 2 cups spinach or kale, chopped
- Fresh parsley for garnish

Instructions:

1. Ground turkey, breadcrumbs, Parmesan cheese, egg, minced garlic, dried oregano, salt, and pepper should all be combined in a bowl. Mix until well blended. Make little meatballs and set them aside.
2. Heat the olive oil in a big saucepan over medium heat. Add the celery, carrots, and chopped onion. Sauté the veggies till they get tender.
3. Include the chopped zucchini and minced garlic in the saucepan. Simmer for a further two to three minutes.

4. Add the chicken broth and diced tomatoes. Add the salt, pepper, dried thyme, and dry rosemary and stir. Simmer the soup for a while.
5. Carefully add the turkey meatballs to the soup that is cooking. Cook until the meatballs are well cooked, 10 to 12 minutes.
6. Cook the chopped kale or spinach in the soup for a further two to three minutes, or until the greens have wilted.
7. Taste and adjust seasoning. Spoon the soup into individual bowls, sprinkle with parsley, and serve hot.

13. Shrimp and avocado lettuce wraps

Ingredients:

For the Shrimp:

- 1 pound large shrimp, peeled and deveined
- 2 tablespoons olive oil
- 2 cloves garlic, minced
- 1 teaspoon paprika
- Salt and pepper to taste
- Juice of 1 lime

For the Lettuce Wraps:

- Large lettuce leaves (such as iceberg or butter lettuce)
- 2 avocados, sliced
- 1 cup cherry tomatoes, halved
- 1/2 red onion, thinly sliced
- Fresh cilantro for garnish

For the Lime Yogurt Sauce:

- 1/2 cup Greek yogurt
- Juice of 1 lime
- 1 tablespoon honey
- Salt and pepper to taste

Instructions:

1. Put the shrimp, olive oil, paprika, chopped garlic, salt, pepper, and lime juice in a bowl. For an even coat, toss.
2. Turn the heat up to medium-high in a skillet. Fry the shrimp for two to three minutes on each side, or until they become opaque and pink. Take off the heat.
3. To make the lime yogurt sauce, combine Greek yogurt, lime juice, honey, salt, and pepper in another bowl.
4. Top each lettuce leaf with a few of shrimp to make the lettuce wraps. Add red onion, cherry tomatoes, and sliced avocado on top.

5. Top with fresh cilantro and drizzle with the lime yogurt sauce over the fillings.
6. Present the avocado and shrimp lettuce wraps right away, topped with more lime wedges if preferred.

14. Whole Grain Pasta with Roasted Vegetables and Marinara Sauce

Ingredients:

- 8 oz whole grain pasta (such as penne, fusilli, or spaghetti)
- 2 cups mixed vegetables (such as bell peppers, zucchini, cherry tomatoes, red onion), chopped
- 2 tablespoons olive oil
- Salt and pepper to taste
- 2 cups marinara sauce (store-bought or homemade)
- **Optional toppings:** grated Parmesan cheese, fresh basil leaves, red pepper flakes

Instructions:

1. Set the oven temperature to 400°F, or 200°C. Use aluminum foil or parchment paper to line a baking pan.

2. Place the chopped mixed veggies in a large mixing basin and toss to coat evenly with olive oil, salt, and pepper.
3. Arrange the seasoned veggies on the baking sheet that has been prepared in a single layer.
4. Roast the veggies for 20 to 25 minutes in a preheated oven, tossing them halfway through, or until they are soft and gently browned.
5. Cook the whole grain pasta according to the package directions until it's al dente while the veggies are roasting. After draining, set away.
6. Heat the marinara sauce in a big skillet or saucepan over medium heat until it's thoroughly cooked.
7. Add the veggies to the skillet with the marinara sauce once they have been roasted and cooked. Stirring helps the sauce cover the veggies uniformly.
8. Include the cooked whole grain pasta, veggies, and sauce in the skillet. Make sure the pasta is covered with sauce by stirring to mix.
9. Cook the pasta for a further two to three minutes, or until it is well warm.
10. Turn off the heat and transfer the whole grain pasta to serving dishes or plates along with the marinara sauce and roasted veggies.
11. Garnish with grated Parmesan cheese, fresh basil leaves, and red pepper flakes, if like, and serve right away.

12. Savor this hearty and delectable whole grain pasta with marinara sauce and roasted veggies. It has a rich tomato sauce, savory roasted vegetables, and soft pasta.

15. Grilled Portobello Mushroom Burgers with Sweet Potato Fries

Ingredients:

For the portobello mushroom burgers:
- 4 large portobello mushroom caps
- 2 tablespoons balsamic vinegar
- 2 tablespoons olive oil
- 2 cloves garlic, minced
- 1 teaspoon dried Italian herbs (such as basil, oregano, thyme)
- Salt and pepper to taste
- 4 whole grain burger buns
- **Optional toppings**: lettuce, tomato slices, red onion slices, avocado slices, cheese slices

For the sweet potato fries:

- 2 large sweet potatoes, peeled and cut into fries
- 2 tablespoons olive oil
- 1 teaspoon paprika

- 1 teaspoon garlic powder
- Salt and pepper to taste

Instructions:

1. Turn the heat up to medium-high on your grill.
2. To make a marinade for the portobello mushrooms, combine the balsamic vinegar, olive oil, chopped garlic, dried Italian herbs, salt, and pepper in a small bowl.
3. Take off the stems from the portobello mushroom caps, then use a moist paper towel to carefully clean them. Make sure that every mushroom cap is equally covered with marinade by placing the caps in a shallow dish or resealable plastic bag. For optimal taste, marinate for at least 30 minutes or up to 4 hours in the refrigerator.
4. Make the sweet potato fries while the mushrooms are marinating. Set the oven temperature to 425°F (220°C).
5. Combine the sweet potato fries, olive oil, paprika, garlic powder, salt, and pepper in a big mixing basin and toss until well coated.
6. Arrange the spiced sweet potato fries in a single layer on a parchment paper-lined baking sheet.
7. Bake the sweet potato fries for 25 to 30 minutes in a preheated oven, turning them halfway through, or until they are crispy and golden brown.
8. Grill the marinated portobello mushroom caps on the preheated grill for 4–5 minutes each side, or until they

are soft and have grill marks, while the sweet potato fries are baking.
9. After the mushrooms are done, take them off the grill and give them some time to rest.
10. Use the grill to gently toast the whole grain burger buns for one to two minutes.
11. Place each grilled mushroom cap on top of a toasted burger bun to assemble the portobello mushroom burgers. Top with chosen ingredients, such as cheese slices, avocado slices, tomato slices, red onion slices, and lettuce.
12. Present the baked sweet potato fries beside the grilled portobello mushroom burgers.
13. Savor this flavorful and filling meal that includes crunchy sweet potato fries and juicy grilled portobello mushrooms.

16. Chicken and Vegetables Curry with Brown Rice

Ingredients:

For the Curry

- 1.5 lbs boneless, skinless chicken thighs, cut into bite-sized pieces

- 2 tablespoons curry powder
- 1 teaspoon ground cumin
- 1 teaspoon ground coriander
- 1 teaspoon turmeric
- 1 tablespoon vegetable oil
- 1 large onion, finely chopped
- 3 cloves garlic, minced
- 1 tablespoon ginger, grated
- 1 can (14 oz) coconut milk
- 1 cup chicken broth
- 2 cups mixed vegetables (such as carrots, bell peppers, and peas)
- Salt and pepper to taste
- Fresh cilantro for garnish

For the Brown Rice:

- 1 cup brown rice
- 2 cups water
- 1/2 teaspoon salt

Instructions:

1. Combine the chicken pieces with turmeric, ground cumin, ground coriander, and curry powder in a bowl. Until the chicken is evenly covered, toss.

2. In a big saucepan over medium heat, warm the vegetable oil. Cook the chopped onion until it becomes tender.
3. Add the grated ginger and minced garlic to the saucepan and cook for one more minute.
4. Add the chicken to the saucepan with the seasonings and cook it until it browns all over.
5. Add the chicken broth and coconut milk. After bringing to a simmer, cook for 15 to 20 minutes, or until the chicken is well cooked.
6. After adding the mixed vegetables to the curry, simmer it for a further five to seven minutes, or until the veggies are soft.
7. Add salt and pepper to taste while seasoning the curry.
8. Prepare the brown rice in a separate pot by mixing rice, water, and salt while the curry is boiling. After bringing to a boil, lower the heat, cover, and simmer the rice for 40 to 45 minutes, or until it is soft.
9. Top brown rice with the Chicken and Vegetable Curry. Add fresh cilantro as a garnish.

17. Turkey and Vegetables Kebabs with Couscous

Ingredients:

For the Turkey and Vegetable Kebabs:

- 1 pound ground turkey
- 1 tablespoon olive oil
- 2 cloves garlic, minced
- 1 teaspoon ground cumin
- 1 teaspoon paprika
- Salt and pepper to taste
- 1 zucchini, cut into chunks
- 1 bell pepper, cut into chunks
- 1 red onion, cut into wedges
- Cherry tomatoes

For the Couscous:

- 1 cup couscous
- 1 cup vegetable or chicken broth
- 1 tablespoon olive oil
- Salt and pepper to taste
- Fresh parsley for garnish

Instructions:

1. Turn the heat up to medium-high on the grill or grill pan.
2. Combine ground turkey, olive oil, minced garlic, paprika, ground cumin, and salt & pepper in a bowl.

Shape tiny amounts of the mixture into the shape of kebabs.
3. Thread bell pepper, red onion, zucchini, and cherry tomatoes in alternate rows with the turkey kebabs.
4. Cook the kebabs on the grill for 5 to 7 minutes on each side, or until the veggies are gently browned and the turkey is cooked through.
5. Get the couscous ready while the kebabs are roasting. Heat the broth in a saucepan until it boils. Add the couscous, cover, and turn off the heat. After five minutes, fluff it with a fork. Add a drizzle of olive oil and season with pepper and salt.
6. Arrange the couscous over the Turkey and Vegetable Kebabs. Add fresh parsley as a garnish.
7. Savor your tasty, high-protein dinner!

18. Vegetable and Tofu Sushi Rolls

Ingredients:

For the Sushi Rice:

- 2 cups sushi rice
- 2 1/2 cups water
- 1/3 cup rice vinegar

- 3 tablespoons sugar
- 1 teaspoon salt

For the Sushi Filling:

- 1 block firm tofu, pressed and cut into strips
- 1 cucumber, julienned
- 1 carrot, julienned
- 1 avocado, sliced
- Nori (seaweed) sheets
- Soy sauce for serving
- Pickled ginger and wasabi (optional)

Instructions:

1. Run cold water over the sushi rice until it flows clear. Follow the directions on the box to cook the rice.
2. Combine rice vinegar, sugar, and salt in a small pot. Cook the sugar over low heat until it melts. After the rice has cooked, pour it into a big basin and whisk in the vinegar mixture very slowly. Let the rice cool until it reaches room temperature.
3. On a level surface, place a bamboo sushi rolling mat. Arrange a nori sheet on the mat, shiny side down.
4. Evenly cover the nori with a thin coating of sushi rice, leaving about half an inch at the top edge. Wet your hands to prevent sticking.

5. Place the avocado, cucumber, carrot, and tofu strips along the rice's lower border.
6. To form the roll, gently press the edge of the bamboo mat nearest the filling up and roll it over the ingredients. Keep rolling until you get to the nori's exposed edge. To seal the roll, dab the edge with a little water and press.
7. Wet it gently with a sharp knife and cut the roll into bite-sized pieces.
8. Proceed with the other ingredients in the same manner.
9. Present the tofu and vegetable sushi rolls beside soy sauce. If desired, garnish with wasabi and pickled ginger.

19. Greek-Style Chicken Pitas with Tzatziki Sauce

Ingredients:

For the Greek-style chicken:

- 1 lb boneless, skinless chicken breasts, sliced into thin strips
- 2 tablespoons olive oil
- 2 cloves garlic, minced
- 1 teaspoon dried oregano
- 1/2 teaspoon dried thyme

- Salt and pepper to taste

For the tzatziki sauce:

- 1 cup Greek yogurt
- 1/2 cucumber, grated and squeezed to remove excess moisture
- 1 clove garlic, minced
- 1 tablespoon lemon juice
- 1 tablespoon fresh dill, chopped (or 1 teaspoon dried dill)
- Salt and pepper to taste

For serving:

- Whole wheat pita bread
- Sliced tomatoes
- Sliced red onion
- Lettuce leaves
- **Optional toppings:** crumbled feta cheese, Kalamata olives, chopped fresh parsley

Instructions:

1. Place the cut chicken breasts in a mixing bowl and add the olive oil, minced garlic, salt, pepper, dried thyme, and dried oregano. Toss until the marinade coats the

chicken evenly. For optimal taste, marinate for at least 30 minutes or up to 4 hours in the refrigerator.

2. Make the tzatziki sauce while the chicken is marinating. Greek yogurt, grated cucumber, minced garlic, lemon juice, chopped dill, salt, and pepper should all be combined in a different mixing dish. Mix well until fully incorporated. If necessary, taste and adjust the seasoning. Keep chilled and covered until you're ready to serve.

3. Turn the heat up to medium-high in a skillet or grill pan. The marinated chicken strips should be added in a single layer once heated. Cook, tossing periodically, until the chicken is cooked through and has a golden brown exterior, 5 to 7 minutes.

4. Follow the directions on the package to reheat the whole wheat pita bread in the oven or on the stovetop while the chicken cooks.

5. Top each hot pita bread with a heaping tablespoon of tzatziki sauce to construct the Greek-style chicken pitas.

6. Arrange cooked chicken pieces, sliced red onion, tomatoes, and lettuce leaves on top of the tzatziki sauce.

7. If preferred, garnish with extra ingredients such chopped fresh parsley, Kalamata olives, and crumbled feta cheese.

8. To create a pocket, fold the pita bread over the filling or roll it up like a wrap.

9. Present the Greek-style chicken pitas right away, and savor the delicious fusion of fresh veggies, creamy tzatziki sauce, and soft chicken.

20. Quinoa and Black Bean Stuffed Bell Peppers

Ingredients:

- 4 large bell peppers, halved and seeds removed
- 1 cup quinoa, cooked according to package instructions
- 1 can (15 oz) black beans, drained and rinsed
- 1 cup corn kernels (fresh or thawed if frozen)
- 1 cup diced tomatoes
- 1 cup shredded cheese (cheddar, Monterey Jack, or your choice)
- 1 teaspoon ground cumin
- 1 teaspoon chili powder
- 1/2 teaspoon garlic powder
- Salt and pepper to taste
- Fresh cilantro or parsley for garnish

Instructions:

1. Turn the oven on to 375°F, or 190°C.

2. Put the cooked quinoa, black beans, corn, diced tomatoes, shredded cheese, chili powder, garlic powder, ground cumin, salt, and pepper in a big mixing bowl. Blend well.
3. Gently press the quinoa and black bean mixture into each side of the bell pepper.
4. Transfer the filled bell peppers to an ovenproof plate.
5. Bake the dish for 25 to 30 minutes, or until the peppers are soft, covered with aluminum foil.
6. Take off the foil and bake for a further five to ten minutes, or until the cheese has melted and the tops have begun to brown.
7. Before serving, sprinkle some fresh parsley or cilantro on top of the filled bell peppers.
8. Savor the rich and nourishing taste of your black bean and quinoa-stuffed bell peppers!

CHAPTER SIX

EASY AND DELICIOUS DINNER RECIPES FOR MANAGING STAGE 4 BREAST CANCER

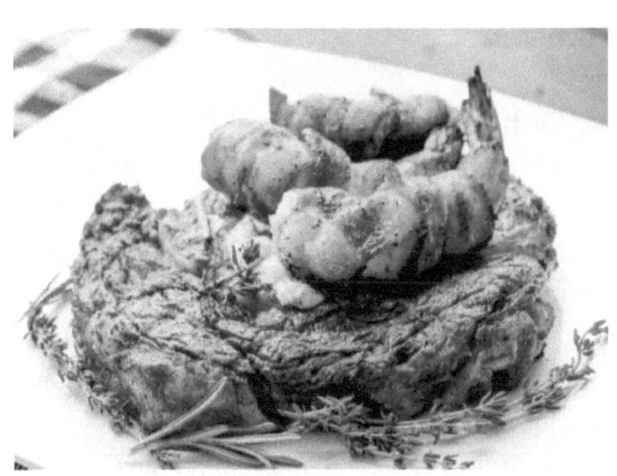

1. Grilled Salmon with Quinoa and Steamed Vegetables

Ingredients:

- 4 salmon filets
- 1 cup quinoa
- 2 cups water or vegetable broth
- Assorted vegetables (such as broccoli, carrots, bell peppers)
- Olive oil
- Salt and pepper to taste
- Lemon wedges for garnish

Instructions:

1. Turn the heat up to medium-high on your grill.
2. Use a fine-mesh strainer to rinse the quinoa in cold water.
3. Put the quinoa and the vegetable broth or water in a medium pot. After bringing to a boil, lower the heat to a simmer, cover, and cook the quinoa for 15 to 20 minutes, or until it is tender and the liquid has been absorbed. Using a fork, fluff and set aside.
4. Prepare the veggies while the quinoa cooks. The various veggies should be cleaned and chopped into bite-sized pieces.

5. Put the veggies on a steaming tray or steamer basket.
6. Steam the veggies for five to seven minutes, or until they are crisp but still tender, over boiling water. Take off the heat and place aside.
7. In the meantime, use paper towels to pat the salmon filets dry and give them a quick olive oil brushing. To taste, add salt and pepper for seasoning.
8. Cook the salmon filets for 4–5 minutes on each side on a hot grill, or until they are cooked through and readily flake with a fork.
9. After the salmon is done, take it off the grill and give it some time to rest.
10. Distribute the cooked quinoa among plates for serving. Add steamed veggies and grilled salmon filets on top.
11. Add some lemon wedges as a garnish and serve right away.

2. Vegetable Stir-Fry with Tofu and Brown Rice

Ingredients:

- 1 block (14 oz) firm tofu, drained and pressed
- 2 tablespoons soy sauce or tamari
- 2 tablespoons sesame oil, divided

- 2 cloves garlic, minced
- 1 tablespoon ginger, minced
- Assorted vegetables (such as bell peppers, broccoli, carrots, snap peas)
- Cooked brown rice
- Salt and pepper to taste
- **Optional toppings:** sliced green onions, sesame seeds, chopped cilantro

Instructions:

1. To begin, press the tofu by sandwiching it between two fresh kitchen towels or paper towels. To press out extra moisture, place a heavy object—like a stack of plates or a cast-iron skillet—on top of the tofu and let it sit for 15 to 30 minutes. Press the tofu and cut it into pieces.
2. Combine the soy sauce or tamari and 1 tablespoon of sesame oil in a small dish. After coating the tofu cubes equally, toss them in the marinade and let them marinate for ten to fifteen minutes.
3. In a large pan or wok, heat the remaining tablespoon of sesame oil over medium-high heat. Ginger and garlic should be added and sautéed for one to two minutes, or until aromatic.
4. Transfer the tofu cubes that have marinated to the pan, setting aside any extra marinade. Stirring periodically, cook the tofu for 5 to 7 minutes, or until golden brown

and crispy on both sides. After taking the tofu out of the skillet, set it aside.

5. Add the various veggies to the same skillet. Stir-fry the veggies for five to seven minutes, or until they are crisp-tender.

6. Add the cooked tofu and veggies back to the skillet. Coat the tofu and veggies evenly by pouring the leftover marinade over them and tossing. Simmer for a further two to three minutes, or until the sauce has somewhat thickened.

7. Add salt and pepper to taste and season the stir-fry.

8. Combine the cooked brown rice with the veggie stir-fry.

9. Add optional garnishes like chopped cilantro, sesame seeds, and sliced green onions.

10. Savor this flavorful and nutrient-dense vegetable stir-fry for a filling lunch or dinner with brown rice and tofu.

3. Turkey and Vegetable Chili with Whole Grain Cornbread

Ingredients:

For the Turkey and Vegetable Chili:

- 1 lb ground turkey
- 1 onion, diced
- 2 cloves garlic, minced
- 1 bell pepper, diced
- 1 zucchini, diced
- 1 carrot, diced
- 1 can (14 oz) diced tomatoes
- 1 can (15 oz) kidney beans, drained and rinsed
- 1 can (15 oz) black beans, drained and rinsed
- 2 tablespoons tomato paste
- 2 cups low-sodium chicken or vegetable broth
- 1 tablespoon chili powder
- 1 teaspoon ground cumin
- 1 teaspoon paprika
- Salt and pepper to taste
- Olive oil for cooking

For the Whole Grain Cornbread:

- 1 cup whole grain cornmeal
- 1 cup whole wheat flour
- 1 tablespoon baking powder
- 1/2 teaspoon salt
- 1 cup milk (dairy or plant-based)
- 1/4 cup honey or maple syrup
- 1/4 cup unsweetened applesauce
- 2 eggs
- 2 tablespoons melted butter or olive oil

Instructions:

For the Turkey and Vegetable Chili:

1. In a big saucepan or Dutch oven, warm a thin layer of olive oil over medium heat. Cook for approximately five minutes, or until the chopped onion is tender.
2. Add the minced garlic and stir until fragrant, about 1 more minute.
3. After adding the ground turkey to the saucepan and breaking it up with a spoon, simmer it until it is well cooked and browned.
4. Add the chopped bell pepper, carrot, and zucchini. Cook, stirring, for 5 to 7 minutes, or until the veggies start to soften.
5. Fill the saucepan with the chopped tomatoes, black beans, kidney beans, tomato paste, chicken or vegetable broth, paprika, ground cumin, chili powder, and salt and pepper. Mix everything together.
6. Simmer the chili for a short while before turning down the heat. To enable the flavors to melt together, cover and simmer for at least 30 minutes, stirring from time to time.
7. Make the whole grain cornbread while the chili is boiling.

For the Whole Grain Cornbread:

1. Set the oven temperature to 375°F, or 190°C. A 9 × 9-inch baking dish should be lined with parchment paper or greased.
2. Combine the whole grain cornmeal, whole wheat flour, baking powder, and salt in a large mixing basin.
3. Combine the milk, eggs, melted butter or olive oil, honey or maple syrup, and unsweetened applesauce in another bowl.
4. Add the liquid mixture to the dry mixture and whisk just until blended. Take caution not to blend too much.
5. Transfer the cornbread mixture into the ready baking dish and use a spatula to level the top.
6. Bake for 20 to 25 minutes in a preheated oven, or until a toothpick inserted into the center comes out clean and the cornbread is golden brown.
7. Before slicing, take the cornbread out of the oven and allow it to cool somewhat.

To Serve:

1. Spoon the veggie and turkey chili into individual bowls.
2. Present the chili with pieces of whole grain cornbread on the side.

3. Savor this filling and healthy dish, which consists of tasty turkey and vegetable chili served with healthy whole grain cornbread.

4. Lentil Soup with Mixed Greens Salad

Ingredients:

For the Lentil Soup:

- 1 cup dried green or brown lentils, rinsed and drained
- 1 onion, finely chopped
- 2 carrots, diced
- 2 celery stalks, diced
- 3 cloves garlic, minced
- 1 can (14 oz) diced tomatoes
- 6 cups vegetable broth
- 1 teaspoon ground cumin
- 1 teaspoon ground coriander
- 1 teaspoon smoked paprika
- Salt and pepper to taste
- 2 tablespoons olive oil
- Fresh lemon wedges for serving

For the Mixed Greens Salad:

- Mixed salad greens (lettuce, spinach, arugula, etc.)
- Cherry tomatoes, halved
- Cucumber, sliced
- Red onion, thinly sliced
- Balsamic vinaigrette dressing

Instructions:

For the Lentil Soup:

1. Heat the olive oil in a big saucepan over medium heat. Add the chopped celery, carrots, and onion. Sauté the veggies till they get tender.
2. Cook the minced garlic for an extra minute after adding it.
3. Add the lentils, diced tomatoes, smoked paprika, ground cumin, ground coriander, and vegetable broth. Season with salt and pepper. Heat the soup until it boils.
4. Once the lentils are soft, reduce heat, cover, and simmer for 25 to 30 minutes.
5. Taste and adjust seasoning. Warm up the lentil soup and drizzle it with freshly squeezed lemon juice.

For the Mixed Greens Salad:

1. Combine red onion, cucumber, cherry tomatoes, and mixed salad greens in a big bowl.

2. Gently toss the salad to coat after drizzling it with balsamic vinaigrette dressing.
3. Present the mixed greens salad with the lentil soup.

5. Baked Chicken Breast with Roasted Sweet Potatoes and Broccoli

Ingredients:

For the Baked Chicken Breast:

- 4 boneless, skinless chicken breasts
- 2 tablespoons olive oil
- 2 cloves garlic, minced
- 1 teaspoon dried thyme
- 1 teaspoon dried rosemary
- Salt and pepper to taste

For the Roasted Sweet Potatoes:

- 2 large sweet potatoes, peeled and diced
- 2 tablespoons olive oil
- 1 teaspoon paprika
- 1/2 teaspoon garlic powder
- Salt and pepper to taste

For the Roasted Broccoli:

- 2 heads broccoli, cut into florets
- 2 tablespoons olive oil
- 2 cloves garlic, minced
- Salt and pepper to taste

Instructions:

1. Set the oven temperature to 400°F, or 200°C. Use aluminum foil or parchment paper to line a baking pan.
2. To make a marinade for the chicken breasts, combine the olive oil, minced garlic, dried thyme, dried rosemary, salt, and pepper in a small dish.
3. Transfer the chicken breasts to the baking sheet that has been ready. Apply the marinade to each chicken breast, being careful to coat it equally on both sides.
4. Evenly coat the diced sweet potatoes in a separate mixing dish using a mixture of olive oil, paprika, garlic powder, salt, and pepper. On one side of the baking sheet, arrange the sweet potatoes in a single layer.
5. Coat the broccoli florets equally with olive oil, minced garlic, salt, and pepper in the same mixing bowl. On the other side of the baking sheet, arrange the broccoli in a single layer.
6. Put the baking sheet in the preheated oven and bake for 25 to 30 minutes, or until the sweet potatoes and broccoli are soft and lightly browned and the chicken is cooked through and reaches an internal temperature of

165°F (74°C). Stir the veggies midway during the baking time.
7. Take the baking sheet out of the oven once it has cooked.
8. Present the roasted sweet potatoes and broccoli with the baked chicken breasts.
9. Savor this filling and healthy dish that consists of tasty roasted sweet potatoes and broccoli combined with a soft baked chicken breast.

6. Shrimp and Vegetable Skewers with Couscous

Ingredients:

For the Shrimp and Vegetable Skewers:

- 1 pound large shrimp, peeled and deveined
- 1 zucchini, sliced into rounds
- 1 bell pepper, cut into chunks
- 1 red onion, cut into wedges
- Cherry tomatoes
- 2 tablespoons olive oil
- 2 cloves garlic, minced
- 1 teaspoon paprika
- 1 teaspoon dried oregano

- Salt and pepper to taste
- Lemon wedges for serving

For the Couscous:

- 1 cup couscous
- 1 cup vegetable or chicken broth
- 1 tablespoon olive oil
- Salt and pepper to taste
- Fresh parsley for garnish

Instructions:

For the Shrimp and Vegetable Skewers:

1. Turn the heat up to medium-high on the grill or grill pan.
2. Put the shrimp, bell pepper pieces, zucchini slices, red onion wedges, and cherry tomatoes in a bowl.
3. Combine olive oil, dried oregano, paprika, minced garlic, salt, and pepper in a small bowl. Pour this mixture over the veggies and shrimp, stirring to coat well.
4. Thread the veggies and shrimp onto skewers in an alternate pattern.
5. Grill the skewers for two to three minutes on each side, or until the shrimp turn opaque and pink.
6. Take the skewers from the grill and give them a quick spritz of lemon juice.

For the Couscous:

1. Bring the broth to a boil in a saucepan. Add the couscous, cover, and turn off the heat. After five minutes, fluff it with a fork.
2. Add salt and pepper to the cooked couscous and drizzle with olive oil. Gently toss to mix.
3. Place a bed of couscous over the shrimp and veggie skewers. Add fresh parsley as a garnish.

7. Spaghetti Squash with Marinara Sauce and Turkey Meatballs

Ingredients:

For the Spaghetti Squash:

- 1 spaghetti squash
- Olive oil
- Salt and pepper to taste

For the Turkey Meatballs:

- 1 lb ground turkey

- 1/4 cup breadcrumbs (whole wheat or gluten-free)
- 1/4 cup grated Parmesan cheese
- 1 egg
- 2 cloves garlic, minced
- 1 teaspoon dried basil
- 1 teaspoon dried oregano
- Salt and pepper to taste

For the Marinara Sauce:

- 1 can (14 oz) crushed tomatoes
- 2 cloves garlic, minced
- 1 teaspoon dried basil
- 1 teaspoon dried oregano
- Salt and pepper to taste

Instructions:

1. Set the oven temperature to 400°F, or 200°C. Use parchment paper to line a baking sheet.
2. Cut the spaghetti squash in half lengthwise, then use a spoon to remove the seeds and stringy parts. Season the squash with salt and pepper and drizzle it with olive oil on the sliced sides.
3. Arrange the squash halves on the baking sheet that has been prepared, cut side down. Squash should be roasted in a preheated oven for 40 to 50 minutes, or until the flesh is fork-tender.

4. Make the turkey meatballs while the squash roasts. Ground turkey, breadcrumbs, egg, grated Parmesan cheese, dried oregano, dried basil, and salt and pepper should all be combined in a mixing dish. Blend until well blended.
5. Using the turkey mixture, form meatballs with a diameter of approximately one inch.
6. In a big skillet over medium heat, pour some olive oil. When the meatballs are cooked through and have browned on both sides, add them to the skillet and simmer for 8 to 10 minutes, flipping them over regularly. After taking the meatballs out of the skillet, set them aside.
7. If necessary, add a little extra olive oil to the same skillet. Cook the minced garlic for one to two minutes, or until it becomes aromatic.
8. Add the salt, pepper, dried oregano, dry basil, and smashed tomatoes. To enable the flavors to mingle, bring the sauce to a simmer and cook, stirring regularly, for 10 to 15 minutes.
9. After roasting, scrape the spaghetti squash's flesh into strands with a fork.
10. Distribute the spaghetti squash strands among plates for serving. Add the turkey meatballs and marinara sauce over top.
11. If preferred, garnish with chopped fresh basil and grated Parmesan cheese.

12. Savor this flavorful and filling turkey meatball with marinara sauce spaghetti squash for a hearty supper.

8. Black Bean and Vegetable Enchiladas with Avocado Salad

Ingredients:

For the Black Bean and Vegetable Enchiladas:

- 1 tablespoon olive oil
- 1 onion, diced
- 2 cloves garlic, minced
- 1 bell pepper, diced
- 1 zucchini, diced
- 1 cup corn kernels (fresh, canned, or frozen)
- 1 can (15 oz) black beans, drained and rinsed
- 1 teaspoon ground cumin
- 1 teaspoon chili powder
- Salt and pepper to taste
- 8 whole wheat or corn tortillas
- 1 can (15 oz) enchilada sauce
- 1 cup shredded cheese (cheddar, Monterey Jack, or a blend)

For the Avocado Salad:

- 2 ripe avocados, diced
- 1 tomato, diced
- 1/4 cup red onion, diced
- 1/4 cup cilantro, chopped
- 1 lime, juiced
- Salt and pepper to taste

Instructions:

For the Black Bean and Vegetable Enchiladas:

1. Set the oven temperature to 375°F, or 190°C. Apply olive oil grease to a 9 x 13-inch baking dish.
2. In a big pan over medium heat, warm the olive oil. Cook for approximately five minutes, or until the chopped onion is tender.
3. Fill the skillet with the diced bell pepper, diced zucchini, diced garlic, and corn kernels. Simmer the veggies for five to seven minutes, or until they are soft.
4. Add the chili powder, ground cumin, black beans, salt, and pepper. For complete heating, cook for a further two to three minutes. Take off the heat and place aside.
5. To make the tortillas malleable, reheat them as directed on the box.
6. Fill each tortilla with a heaping spoonful of the black bean and veggie mixture. After rolling the tortillas, put

them seam side down in the baking dish that has been ready.
7. Evenly cover the rolled tortillas with the enchilada sauce by pouring it over them.
8. Top the enchiladas with the cheese that has been shredded.
9. Bake the dish in the preheated oven for 20 to 25 minutes, or until the cheese is bubbling and melted, covered with aluminum foil.
10. Take off the foil and bake for a further five minutes, or until the cheese is gently browned.

For the Avocado Salad:

1. Diced avocados, diced tomatoes, diced red onions, chopped cilantro, lime juice, salt, and pepper should all be combined in a mixing dish. Toss gently until well blended.
2. Present the heated black bean and veggie enchiladas with avocado salad on top.
3. Savor this filling and tasty dish that consists of creamy avocado salad and enchiladas with a delectable filling of black beans and veggies.

9. Baked Tilapia with Lemon Herb Sauce and Quinoa Pilaf

Ingredients:

For the Baked Tilapia:

- 4 tilapia filets
- 2 tablespoons olive oil
- 2 cloves garlic, minced
- 1 lemon, thinly sliced
- Salt and pepper to taste

For the Lemon Herb Sauce:

- 1/4 cup fresh lemon juice
- 2 tablespoons olive oil
- 2 cloves garlic, minced
- 1 tablespoon chopped fresh parsley
- 1 tablespoon chopped fresh dill
- Salt and pepper to taste

For the Quinoa Pilaf:

- 1 cup quinoa, rinsed
- 2 cups low-sodium chicken or vegetable broth
- 1 tablespoon olive oil
- 1 onion, diced
- 2 cloves garlic, minced
- 1 carrot, diced

- 1 bell pepper, diced
- 1/4 cup chopped fresh parsley
- Salt and pepper to taste

Instructions:

For the Baked Tilapia:

1. Set the oven temperature to 400°F, or 200°C. Use aluminum foil or parchment paper to line a baking pan.
2. Using paper towels, pat the tilapia filets dry before arranging them on the baking pan.
3. Combine the olive oil, salt, pepper, and chopped garlic in a small bowl. Drizzle the blend onto the filets of tilapia.
4. Top each tilapia filet with a slice of lemon.
5. Bake the tilapia for ten to twelve minutes, or until it is opaque and flakes readily with a fork, in the preheated oven.

For the Lemon Herb Sauce:

1. Combine the olive oil, minced garlic, chopped parsley, chopped dill, fresh lemon juice, salt, and pepper in a small saucepan.
2. Turn up the heat to medium and whisk regularly to fully heat the sauce. Take off the heat and place aside.

For the Quinoa Pilaf:

1. Heat the vegetable or chicken broth in a medium pot until it boils.
2. Add the boiling broth to the washed quinoa. Once the quinoa is cooked and the liquid has been absorbed, reduce the heat to low, cover, and simmer for 15 to 20 minutes.
3. In a large pan over medium heat, warm the olive oil while the quinoa cooks. To the pan, add the chopped bell pepper, diced onion, diced carrot, and minced garlic. Simmer the veggies for five to seven minutes, or until they are soft.
4. After the quinoa is done, add it to the skillet with the sautéed veggies and fluff it up with a fork. Mix everything together.
5. Top the quinoa pilaf with chopped parsley and season with salt and pepper to taste. Mix well until well blended.

To Serve:

1. Distribute the pilaf of quinoa among serving dishes.
2. Top each serving of quinoa pilaf with a baked tilapia filet.
3. Cover the tilapia filets with a drizzle of the lemon-herb sauce.

4. If preferred, garnish with more finely chopped fresh parsley and dill.
5. Savor this tasty and light dinner of quinoa pilaf and baked filets with lemon herb sauce.

10. Eggplant Parmesan with Whole Wheat Pasta

Ingredients:

For the Eggplant Parmesan:

- 2 large eggplants, sliced into 1/2-inch rounds
- Salt
- 2 cups whole wheat breadcrumbs
- 1 cup grated Parmesan cheese
- 2 eggs, beaten
- Olive oil for frying
- 2 cups marinara sauce
- 1 cup shredded mozzarella cheese
- Fresh basil leaves for garnish

For the Whole Wheat Pasta:

- 8 ounces whole wheat spaghetti or pasta of your choice
- Salt

Instructions:

For the Eggplant Parmesan:

1. After putting the eggplant slices in a strainer, liberally salt them. Give them a half hour or so to drain off any extra moisture.
2. Make the breadcrumb mixture in the interim. Combine the grated Parmesan cheese and whole wheat breadcrumbs in a shallow dish.
3. After 30 minutes, use paper towels to wipe dry the eggplant slices after rinsing them in cold water.
4. Coat each eggplant slice in the breadcrumb mixture and gently press to adhere after dipping it into the beaten eggs.
5. In a big skillet set over medium-high heat, warm up the olive oil. Fry the breaded eggplant slices in batches for 3–4 minutes on each side, or until golden brown and crispy on all sides. Empty any extra oil by transferring to a dish covered with paper towels.
6. Set the oven's temperature to 375°F (190°C).
7. Lightly coat the bottom of a 9 x 13-inch baking dish with marinara sauce. Over the sauce, arrange half of the fried eggplant slices in a single layer. Sprinkle half of the shredded mozzarella cheese and extra marinara sauce on top.

8. Continue with the leftover marinara sauce, shredded mozzarella cheese, and eggplant pieces.
9. Bake for 25 to 30 minutes, or until the cheese is bubbling and melted, in a preheated oven.

For the Whole Wheat Pasta:

1. Boil a big pot of salted water while the eggplant Parmesan is baking. Cook the whole wheat pasta until al dente, following the directions on the package.
2. Place the cooked pasta back into the pot after draining.

To Serve:

1. Spoon cooked whole wheat pasta onto each of the serving dishes.
2. Add some eggplant Parmesan on the top of each plate of pasta.
3. Add fresh basil leaves as a garnish.
4. Savor this flavorful and nourishing dish of whole wheat pasta with eggplant parmesan.

11. Thai Coconut Curry with Tofu and Jasmine Rice

Ingredients:

- 1 block (about 14 oz) of extra-firm tofu, drained and cubed
- 1 tablespoon vegetable oil
- 1 small onion, finely chopped
- 2 cloves garlic, minced
- 1 red bell pepper, sliced
- 1 yellow bell pepper, sliced
- 1 cup broccoli florets
- 1 can (13.5 oz) coconut milk
- 2 tablespoons red curry paste
- 1 tablespoon soy sauce (or tamari for gluten-free option)
- 1 tablespoon brown sugar
- 1 tablespoon lime juice
- Salt and pepper to taste
- Fresh cilantro, chopped, for garnish
- Cooked jasmine rice, for serving

Instructions:

1. In a large skillet or wok, heat the vegetable oil over medium-high heat. Add the cubed tofu and heat for 5 to 7 minutes, or until golden brown on both sides. After taking the tofu out of the skillet, set it aside.
2. Add the minced garlic and chopped onion to the same skillet, and add a little extra oil if necessary. Sauté the onion for two to three minutes, or until it is aromatic and transparent.

3. Include the broccoli florets and the sliced red and yellow bell peppers in the skillet. Simmer for a further 3–4 minutes, or until the veggies are starting to soften.
4. Add the coconut milk and mix in the lime juice, brown sugar, soy sauce, and red curry paste. After giving everything a good stir, reduce the heat to a simmer.
5. Return the fried tofu to the skillet once the curry sauce has simmered. Toss to distribute the sauce over the tofu and veggies. Simmer the curry for a further five to seven minutes, stirring now and again, until the flavors blend together and the sauce gets a little thicker.
6. To taste, add salt and pepper for seasoning.
7. Spoon the cooked jasmine rice over the Thai coconut curry. Before serving, add some freshly cut cilantro as a garnish.

12. Stuffed Bell Peppers with Quinoa, Black Beans, and Cheese

Ingredients:

- 4 large bell peppers (any color), halved and seeds removed
- 1 cup quinoa, rinsed
- 1 can (15 oz) black beans, drained and rinsed

- 1 cup corn kernels (fresh, frozen, or canned)
- 1 cup diced tomatoes (fresh or canned)
- 1 small onion, finely chopped
- 2 cloves garlic, minced
- 1 teaspoon ground cumin
- 1 teaspoon chili powder
- Salt and pepper to taste
- 1 cup shredded cheese (cheddar, Monterey Jack, or Mexican blend)
- Fresh cilantro, chopped, for garnish

Instructions:

1. Set the oven temperature to 375°F, or 190°C.
2. Place two cups of water in a medium pot and heat to a boil. After adding the quinoa, turn down the heat to low, cover, and simmer until the quinoa is tender and the water has been absorbed, about 15 minutes. Take off the heat and use a fork to fluff.
3. The cooked quinoa, black beans, corn kernels, diced tomatoes, chopped onion, minced garlic, ground cumin, chili powder, salt, and pepper should all be combined in a big mixing basin. Mix well to blend.
4. Place the bell pepper halves cut-side up in a baking tray.
5. Gently push down to cram the fillings into each bell pepper half after stuffing it with the quinoa and black bean mixture.

6. Bake the baking dish in the preheated oven for 25 to 30 minutes, or until the bell peppers are soft, covered with aluminum foil.
7. Take off the foil from the baking dish, cover the filled bell peppers with the shredded cheese, and put it back in the oven. Bake for a further five to seven minutes, or until the cheese is bubbling and melted.
8. Take it out of the oven and give it a little time to cool before serving.
9. Before serving, garnish with finely chopped fresh cilantro.

13. Greek-Style Chicken Pitas with Tzatziki Sauce and Greek Salad

Ingredients:

- 4 boneless, skinless chicken breasts
- 2 tablespoons olive oil
- 2 cloves garlic, minced
- 1 teaspoon dried oregano
- 1 teaspoon dried thyme
- Salt and pepper to taste
- 4 whole wheat pitas
- Tzatziki sauce (store-bought or homemade)

- Greek salad ingredients (cucumbers, tomatoes, red onion, Kalamata olives, feta cheese)

Instructions:

1. Combine olive oil, minced garlic, dried thyme, dried oregano, salt, and pepper in a basin to make a marinade.
2. Coat the chicken breasts well with the marinade after adding them. Allow to marinate for at least half an hour, or better yet, overnight.
3. Adjust the heat to medium-high and preheat the grill or grill pan. Cook chicken breasts on the grill for 6–7 minutes on each side, or until they are well cooked and the middle is no longer pink. Take off from the heat and allow it to sit for a little while.
4. Toast the pitas or cook them on the grill while the chicken is resting.
5. Thinly slice the cooked chicken breasts.
6. Spread a sufficient quantity of Tzatziki sauce on each pita to assemble the pitas. Top with Greek salad ingredients and add the cut chicken.
7. Immediately serve by folding the pita over the fillings.

14. Caprese Salad with Grilled Chicken and Whole Grain Bread

Ingredients:

- 2 boneless, skinless chicken breasts
- Salt and pepper to taste
- 2 tablespoons olive oil
- 2 large tomatoes, sliced
- 1 ball fresh mozzarella cheese, sliced
- Fresh basil leaves
- Balsamic glaze, for drizzling (optional)
- 4 slices whole grain bread, toasted

Instructions:

1. Turn the heat up to medium-high on your grill or grill pan.
2. Drizzle some olive oil and season the chicken breasts with salt and pepper.
3. Cook the chicken breasts on the grill for 6 to 8 minutes on each side, or until they are cooked through and no longer have a pink core. Take it out of the grill and let it rest for a few minutes to rest before slicing.
4. As the chicken grills, make the Caprese salad by dividing the mozzarella cheese and tomato slices into two rows on a serving tray.
5. Place a few fresh basil leaves in between the mozzarella and tomato slices.
6. Cut the chicken into thin strips when it has finished cooking and resting.

7. Top the caprese salad with the grilled chicken slices.
8. For extra flavor, drizzle the salad with balsamic glaze, if preferred.
9. Present the grilled chicken and caprese salad with pieces of toasted whole grain bread.

15. Veggie Burgers with Sweet Potato Fries

Veggie Burgers:

Ingredients:

- 1 can (15 oz) black beans, drained and rinsed
- 1 cup cooked quinoa
- 1/2 cup finely chopped onion
- 1/2 cup grated carrot
- 1/4 cup finely chopped bell pepper (any color)
- 2 cloves garlic, minced
- 2 tablespoons chopped fresh parsley
- 1 teaspoon ground cumin
- 1 teaspoon paprika
- Salt and pepper to taste
- 1 tablespoon olive oil (for cooking)

Instructions:

1. Using a fork or potato masher, roughly mash the black beans in a large mixing basin until they are mostly smooth.
2. To the mashed black beans, add the cooked quinoa, ground cumin, paprika, chopped onion, shredded carrot, diced bell pepper, minced garlic, chopped parsley, and salt and pepper. Blend until well blended.
3. Form the ingredients into patties by dividing it into equal sections.
4. In a pan over medium heat, warm the olive oil. The vegetable burger patties should be cooked for 4–5 minutes on each side, or until they are well roasted and golden brown.
5. Top the vegetable burgers with your preferred condiments, lettuce, tomato, and avocado and serve them on whole grain buns.

Sweet Potato Fries:

Ingredients:

- 2 large sweet potatoes, peeled and cut into fries
- 2 tablespoons olive oil
- 1 teaspoon garlic powder
- 1 teaspoon paprika
- Salt and pepper to taste

Instructions:

1. Preheat the oven to 425°F (220°C), and place parchment paper on a baking pan.
2. Toss the sweet potato fries with olive oil, salt, pepper, paprika, and garlic powder in a large mixing basin until well coated.
3. Arrange the seasoned sweet potato fries on the baking sheet that has been ready in a single layer.
4. Bake the fries for 20 to 25 minutes in a preheated oven, turning them over halfway through, or until they are crispy and browned.
5. Present the sweet potato fries as a tasty and wholesome side dish to go with the veggie burgers.

16. Spinach and Feta Stuffed Chicken Breasts with Roasted Vegetables

Spinach and Feta Stuffed Chicken Breasts:

Ingredients:

- 4 boneless, skinless chicken breasts
- 2 cups fresh spinach leaves
- 1/2 cup crumbled feta cheese

- 2 cloves garlic, minced
- 1 tablespoon olive oil
- Salt and pepper to taste
- Toothpicks or kitchen twine

Instructions:

1. Set the oven temperature to 375°F, or 190°C.
2. Make a horizontal pocket in each chicken breast with a sharp knife, taking care not to cut all the way through.
3. Heat the olive oil in a pan over medium heat. Cook the minced garlic for one to two minutes, or until it becomes aromatic.
4. Cook the fresh spinach leaves in the pan for two to three minutes, or until they have wilted.
5. Take the pan off of the burner and let the combination of spinach cool somewhat.
6. Stir in the feta cheese crumbles when it has cooled.
7. Stuff the spinach and feta mixture inside each chicken breast, making sure the filling is held within by tying the holes together with kitchen twine or toothpicks.
8. Add salt and pepper to taste while spicing the filled chicken breasts.
9. Transfer the stuffed chicken breasts to a baking tray, then bake for 25 to 30 minutes in a preheated oven, or until the chicken is well cooked and the middle is no longer pink.

Roasted Vegetables:

Ingredients:

- 4 cups mixed vegetables (such as carrots, bell peppers, zucchini, and red onion), chopped
- 2 tablespoons olive oil
- 1 teaspoon dried Italian seasoning
- Salt and pepper to taste

Instructions:

1. Arrange the chopped mixed veggies on a parchment paper-lined baking sheet.
2. Season the veggies with salt, pepper, and dry Italian spice after drizzling them with olive oil. For an even coat, toss.
3. Roast the veggies, stirring halfway through, in the preheated oven for 20 to 25 minutes, or until they are soft and beginning to caramelize.

Assembly:

1. Take the roasted veggies and chicken breasts out of the oven once they are done.
2. Present the feta and spinach-stuffed chicken breasts with the roasted veggies on the side.

17. Portobello Mushroom Burgers with Mixed Greens Salad

Portobello Mushroom Burgers:

Ingredients:

- 4 large Portobello mushroom caps, stems removed
- 4 whole grain burger buns
- 2 tablespoons balsamic vinegar
- 2 tablespoons soy sauce (or tamari for gluten-free option)
- 2 cloves garlic, minced
- 2 tablespoons olive oil
- Salt and pepper to taste
- **Optional toppings:** sliced tomato, avocado, red onion, lettuce, cheese (vegan or dairy), mustard, mayonnaise

Instructions:

1. To create the marinade, mix together the balsamic vinegar, soy sauce, olive oil, minced garlic, salt, and pepper in a small bowl.

2. Transfer the Portobello mushroom caps to a shallow dish and cover them well with marinade. Allow them to marinade for a minimum of twenty to thirty minutes, rotating them midway.
3. Turn the heat to medium on your grill or grill pan.
4. Grill the marinated Portobello mushroom caps until they are soft and have grill marks, about 4–5 minutes each side.
5. If preferred, toast the burger buns while the mushrooms are cooking.
6. Place each grilled mushroom cap on a burger bun and top with your preferred toppings to assemble the Portobello mushroom burgers.
7. Present right away.

Mixed Greens Salad:

Ingredients:

- 4 cups mixed greens (such as spinach, arugula, kale, or lettuce)
- 1 cup cherry tomatoes, halved
- 1/2 cucumber, sliced
- 1/4 red onion, thinly sliced
- 1/4 cup crumbled feta cheese (optional)
- Balsamic vinaigrette dressing

Instructions:

1. Combine the mixed greens, cherry tomatoes, cucumber slices, red onion slices, and crumbled feta cheese in a large mixing basin.
2. Gently toss the salad to coat after drizzling it with balsamic vinaigrette dressing.
3. As a cool side dish, serve the mixed greens salad with the Portobello mushroom burgers.

18. Teriyaki Glazed Salmon with Brown Rice and Stir-fried Vegetables

Teriyaki Glazed Salmon:

Ingredients:

- 4 salmon filets (about 6 oz each), skin-on or skinless
- 1/4 cup soy sauce
- 2 tablespoons honey or maple syrup
- 2 tablespoons rice vinegar
- 2 cloves garlic, minced
- 1 teaspoon grated ginger
- 1 tablespoon cornstarch (optional, for thickening the sauce)

- Sesame seeds and sliced green onions for garnish (optional)

Instructions:

1. To create the teriyaki sauce, combine the soy sauce, rice vinegar, honey or maple syrup, chopped garlic, and grated ginger in a small bowl.
2. If desired, you may thicken the sauce by adding the cornstarch mixture to the teriyaki sauce mixture after combining it with a tablespoon of water in a separate small bowl. Mix well until fully incorporated.
3. Transfer the salmon filets to a shallow dish or resealable plastic bag, and cover them well with the teriyaki sauce. Let it marinate for a minimum of half an hour or for as long as two hours in the fridge.
4. Set the oven temperature to 200°C, or 400°F.
5. Take the salmon out of the marinade and put it on a parchment paper-lined baking sheet.
6. Bake the salmon for 12 to 15 minutes, or until it's cooked through and flaky, being sure to baste it halfway through with the leftover marinade.
7. When the salmon is done, take it out of the oven and, if you'd like, top it with sliced green onions and sesame seeds.

Brown Rice:

Follow the directions on the package to prepare the brown rice. Generally, you will need two cups of water for each cup of rice. After bringing water to a boil, add rice, cover, and simmer until rice is soft and water is absorbed, around 40 to 45 minutes.

Stir-Fried Vegetables:

Ingredients:

- 2 cups mixed vegetables (such as bell peppers, broccoli, carrots, snap peas, mushrooms, etc.), sliced or chopped
- 2 tablespoons soy sauce
- 1 tablespoon sesame oil
- 2 cloves garlic, minced
- 1 teaspoon grated ginger
- Sesame seeds for garnish (optional)

Instructions:

1. In a large skillet or wok, heat the sesame oil over medium-high heat.
2. Stir-fry the grated ginger and minced garlic for approximately a minute, or until fragrant.
3. Stir-fry the mixed veggies in the pan for 4–5 minutes, or until they are crisp-tender.

4. Drizzle the veggies with soy sauce and toss to cover well. Simmer for one or two more minutes.
5. Take off the heat and, if you'd like, sprinkle with sesame seeds.

Assembly:

1. Present the brown rice and stir-fried veggies with the salmon coated in teriyaki glaze.
2. Drizzle the salmon and rice with any leftover teriyaki sauce from the baking sheet.

19. Baked Falafel with Tahini Sauce and Tabbouleh Salad

Baked Falafel:

Ingredients:

- 1 can (15 oz) chickpeas, drained and rinsed
- 1/2 cup fresh parsley, chopped
- 1/2 cup fresh cilantro, chopped
- 1 small onion, chopped
- 2 cloves garlic, minced
- 1 teaspoon ground cumin
- 1 teaspoon ground coriander

- 1/4 teaspoon cayenne pepper (optional)
- 2 tablespoons all-purpose flour or chickpea flour
- 1 teaspoon baking powder
- Salt and pepper to taste
- Olive oil, for brushing

Instructions:

1. Set the oven to 375°F (190°C) and brush a baking sheet with a little amount of olive oil.
2. Put the chickpeas, flour, baking powder, salt, pepper, cayenne pepper (if using), onion, garlic, parsley, cilantro, cumin, and coriander in a food processor. Pulse the mixture until it's well mixed but has some chunks remaining.
3. Form the falafel mixture into little patties or balls with your hands, then arrange them on the baking sheet that has been ready.
4. Apply a thin layer of olive oil to the falafel's tops.
5. Bake for 20 to 25 minutes in a preheated oven, turning the falafel halfway through, or until it's crispy and golden brown.

Tahini Sauce:

Ingredients:

- 1/4 cup tahini

- 2 tablespoons lemon juice
- 1 clove garlic, minced
- 2-4 tablespoons water
- Salt to taste

Instructions:

1. Combine the tahini, lemon juice, salt, and minced garlic in a small bowl.
2. Add water one tablespoon at a time, gradually, until the sauce has the consistency you want. The sauce ought to be pourable and silky.
3. Taste and, if needed, adjust the seasoning.

Tabbouleh Salad:

Ingredients:

- 1/2 cup bulgur wheat
- 1 cup boiling water
- 1 cup fresh parsley, chopped
- 1/2 cup fresh mint leaves, chopped
- 2 tomatoes, diced
- 1/2 cucumber, diced
- 1/4 cup red onion, finely chopped
- 2 tablespoons lemon juice
- 2 tablespoons olive oil
- Salt and pepper to taste

Instructions:

1. Transfer the bulgur wheat to a heat-resistant bowl and cover it with boiling water. After the bulgur has absorbed the water and become delicate, cover and let it sit for 15 to 20 minutes. Using a fork, fluff.
2. Put the cooked bulgur wheat, diced tomatoes, diced cucumber, finely sliced red onion, chopped parsley, and chopped mint leaves in a big bowl.
3. Combine the lemon juice, olive oil, salt, and pepper in a small bowl. After adding the dressing to the salad, stir to mix.
4. Taste and, if needed, adjust the seasoning.

Assembly:

1. Present the tabbouleh salad and tahini sauce with the baked falafel.
2. You can choose to serve this with warm wraps or pita bread.

20. Roasted Vegetables and Chickpea Buddha Bowls with Quinoa and Tahini Dressing

Ingredients:

For Roasted Vegetables and Chickpeas:

- 2 cups mixed vegetables (such as bell peppers, zucchini, carrots, broccoli, etc.), chopped
- 1 can (15 oz) chickpeas, drained and rinsed
- 2 tablespoons olive oil
- 1 teaspoon garlic powder
- 1 teaspoon smoked paprika
- Salt and pepper to taste

For Quinoa:

- 1 cup quinoa, rinsed
- 2 cups water or vegetable broth
- Salt to taste

For Tahini Dressing:

- 1/4 cup tahini
- 2 tablespoons lemon juice
- 2 tablespoons water
- 1 clove garlic, minced
- 1/2 teaspoon ground cumin
- Salt and pepper to taste

Optional toppings:

- Fresh parsley or cilantro, chopped
- Sesame seeds

Instructions:

Roasted Vegetables and Chickpeas:

1. Preheat the oven to 400°F (200°C) and place parchment paper on a baking pan.
2. Combine the mixed veggies and chickpeas in a big bowl and toss to cover them equally with the olive oil, smoked paprika, garlic powder, and salt and pepper.
3. Arrange the chickpeas and seasoned veggies in a single layer on the baking sheet that has been ready.
4. Roast, stirring halfway through cooking, in a preheated oven for 20 to 25 minutes, or until the veggies are soft and the chickpeas are crispy.

For Quinoa:

1. Place the washed quinoa and vegetable broth or water in a saucepan.
2. After bringing to a boil, lower the heat to a simmer, cover, and cook the quinoa for 15 to 20 minutes, or until it is tender and the liquid has been absorbed.
3. Turn off the heat and leave it covered for five minutes. Use a fork to fluff before serving.

For Tahini Dressing:

Until smooth and creamy, mix together tahini, lemon juice, water, ground cumin, minced garlic, salt, and pepper in a small bowl. To get the consistency you want, add extra water if necessary.

Assembly:

1. Spoon cooked quinoa into each of the serving dishes.
2. Add chickpeas and roasted veggies to the top of each bowl.
3. Cover the dishes with a tahini dressing drizzle.
4. If preferred, garnish with sesame seeds and finely chopped fresh parsley or cilantro.
5. Present your delectable Quinoa and Tahini Dressed Roasted Vegetable and Chickpea Buddha Bowls immediately!

CHAPTER SEVEN

QUICK AND EASY SNACKS AND DESSERTS OPTION FOR MANAGING STAGE 4 BREAST CANCER

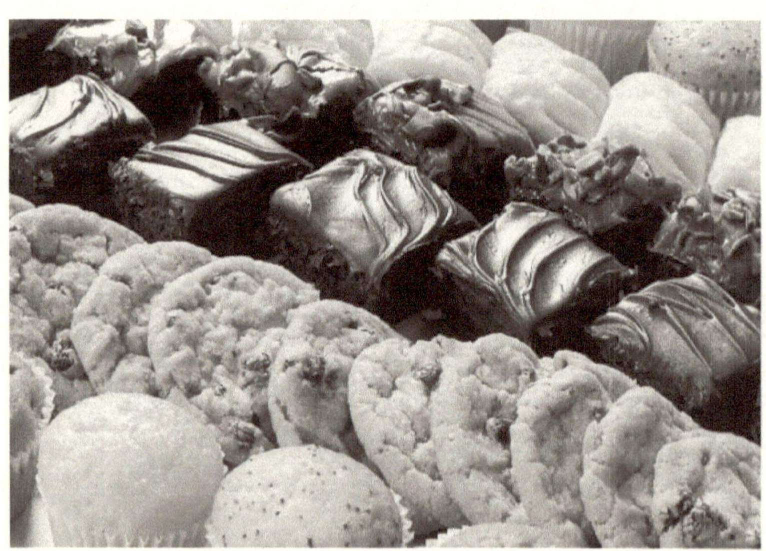

1. Greek Yogurt with Honey and Sliced Almonds

Ingredients:

- 1 cup Greek yogurt (plain or flavored)
- 1 tablespoon honey (adjust to taste)
- 2 tablespoons sliced almonds

Instructions:

1. Transfer the Greek yogurt with a spoon into a serving dish or individual cups.
2. Drizzle the Greek yogurt with honey, adjusting the quantity to suit your desired level of sweetness.
3. Top the yogurt and honey with sliced almonds.
4. Present right away and savor!

2. Fresh Fruit Salad with a Sprinkle of Cinnamon

Ingredients:

- Assorted fresh fruits (such as strawberries, blueberries, pineapple, grapes, kiwi, mango, oranges, etc.), washed, peeled, and chopped as needed
- Ground cinnamon

Instructions:

1. Wash and peel the various fresh fruits (if needed), then slice them into bite-sized pieces.
2. Combine the chopped fruits in a large mixing dish.
3. Depending on your taste, sprinkle ground cinnamon on top of the fruit salad. Start with a little quantity and make adjustments as needed.
4. Toss the fruit salad gently to distribute the cinnamon evenly.
5. Serve immediately or store in the fridge for a wholesome and revitalizing dessert or snack choice.

3. Whole Grain Crackers with Hummus and Sliced Vegetables

Ingredients:

- Whole grain crackers
- Hummus (store-bought or homemade)

- Assorted vegetables (such as carrots, cucumbers, bell peppers, cherry tomatoes, celery, etc.), washed and sliced

Instructions:

1. Arrange the whole grain crackers individually or on a serving tray.
2. Top each cracker with a generous dollop of hummus.
3. Arrange the hummus and crackers on the serving dish, then add the cut veggies.
4. Enjoy your Whole Grain Crackers with Hummus and Sliced Vegetables as a delightful and wholesome appetizer or snack, served right away.

4. Cottage Cheese with Pineapple Chunks

Ingredients:

- 1 cup cottage cheese
- 1/2 cup pineapple chunks (fresh or canned, drained)

Instructions:

1. Place a little amount of cottage cheese in a serving dish.

2. Top the cottage cheese with the pineapple chunks.
3. You may either leave the pineapple and cottage cheese stacked for show, or you can gently mix them together.
4. Enjoy your cottage cheese with pineapple chunks as a filling and healthy snack or as a light meal alternative by serving it right away.

5. Apple Slices with Peanut Butter or Almond Butter

Ingredients:

- 1-2 apples, washed and sliced
- Peanut butter or almond butter

Instructions:

1. After giving the apples a good wash, cut them into rounds or wedges and remove any seeds or stems.
2. Apply almond or peanut butter to each apple slice.
3. Arrange the apple slices on a serving platter with almond or peanut butter.
4. Enjoy your tasty and wholesome apple slices with almond or peanut butter right away as a light dessert or as a healthy snack.

6. Trail Mix with Nuts, Seeds, and Dried Fruit

Ingredients:

- 1 cup mixed nuts (such as almonds, cashews, walnuts, peanuts, etc.), unsalted
- 1/2 cup mixed seeds (such as pumpkin seeds, sunflower seeds, flaxseeds, etc.)
- 1/2 cup dried fruit (such as raisins, cranberries, apricots, dates, etc.)
- **Optional:** 1/4 cup dark chocolate chips or chunks

Instructions:

1. Combine the dried fruit, mixed nuts, and optional dark chocolate pieces or chips in a large mixing dish.
2. Give the ingredients a good stir to distribute them evenly.
3. To make the trail mix easier to carry on the move, transfer it to an airtight container or separate it into individual snack bags.
4. Till you're ready to use it, keep the trail mix in a cold, dry location.

7. Banana Slices with Dark Chocolate Chips

Ingredients:

- 1-2 ripe bananas
- Dark chocolate chips or chunks

Instructions:

1. After peeling, cut the bananas into rounds that are between 1/4 and 1/2 inch thick.
2. Arrange the slices of banana on a tray or dish for serving.
3. Top the banana slices with chunks or chips of dark chocolate.
4. As a wholesome and filling snack or dessert, serve your decadent and delicious banana slices with dark chocolate chips right away.

For a cool frozen treat, you may also freeze the banana slices with dark chocolate chips. Just put the completed banana slices on a baking sheet covered with parchment paper, then freeze until the chocolate sets. After that, move the frozen banana slices to a freezer-safe container and keep them there until you're ready to eat them.

8. Veggie Sticks with Tzatziki Dip

Ingredients:

- Assorted fresh vegetables (such as carrots, cucumbers, bell peppers, celery, cherry tomatoes, etc.), washed and cut into sticks or wedges
- Tzatziki dip (store-bought or homemade)

For Tzatziki Dip:

- 1 cup Greek yogurt
- 1/2 cucumber, grated and drained
- 1-2 cloves garlic, minced
- 1 tablespoon fresh lemon juice
- 1 tablespoon extra virgin olive oil
- 1 tablespoon fresh dill, chopped (or 1 teaspoon dried dill)
- Salt and pepper to taste

Instructions:

For Tzatziki Dip:

1. Greek yogurt, grated and drained cucumber, minced garlic, lemon juice, olive oil, chopped dill, salt, and pepper should all be combined in a bowl. Mix until fully blended.
2. To let the flavors combine, cover and chill the tzatziki dip for at least half an hour.

For Veggie Sticks:

1. Trim and chop a variety of fresh veggies into wedges or sticks.
2. Place the veggie sticks on separate plates or a serving dish.
3. Arrange a bowl of tzatziki dip on each plate's side or in the middle of the platter.
4. Enjoy your Veggie Sticks with Tzatziki Dip as a tasty and nutritious snack or appetizer by serving them right away.

You may modify this recipe to your liking by substituting your preferred veggies and tzatziki dip spices to your own taste. For added taste, you may also add fresh herbs or spices.

9. Rice Cakes with Avocado Mash and Cherry Tomatoes

Ingredients:

- Rice cakes
- 1 ripe avocado
- Cherry tomatoes, halved
- Salt and pepper to taste
- **Optional toppings:** sesame seeds, red pepper flakes, fresh herbs (such as cilantro or parsley)

Instructions:

1. Scoop out the ripe avocado flesh and use a fork to mash it smooth in a small bowl.
2. Add salt and pepper to taste and thoroughly combine with the avocado mash.
3. Top each rice cake with a heaping portion of avocado mash.
4. Place halved cherry tomatoes on top of the avocado mash and gently press them into the avocado.
5. As an optional garnish and flavoring, top the rice cakes with sesame seeds, red pepper flakes, or fresh herbs.
6. Present your mouth watering Rice Cakes accompanied with Avocado Mash and Cherry Tomatoes right away,

and savor them as a healthy and nourishing snack or appetizer.

You are welcome to alter this dish to suit your tastes by adding more ingredients or toppings. For variation, try experimenting with other kinds of rice cakes.

10. Frozen Grapes or Berries

Ingredients:

- Grapes or berries (such as strawberries, blueberries, raspberries, or blackberries)

Instructions:

1. . Wash the grapes or berries thoroughly under cold water and pat them dry with a clean kitchen towel.
2. **For grapes:** Remove the stems and place the grapes in a single layer on a baking sheet lined with parchment paper. Make sure the grapes are not touching each other.
   For berries: Spread the berries in a single layer on a baking sheet lined with parchment paper.
3. Place the baking sheet in the freezer and let the grapes or berries freeze for at least 2-3 hours, or until they are completely frozen.

4. Once frozen, transfer the grapes or berries to an airtight container or freezer bag for storage.
5. Keep the frozen grapes or berries in the freezer until ready to enjoy.

11. Chia Seed Pudding with Berries

Ingredients:

- 1/4 cup chia seeds
- 1 cup milk of your choice (such as almond milk, coconut milk, or dairy milk)
- 1 tablespoon maple syrup or honey (optional, for sweetness)
- 1/2 teaspoon vanilla extract
- Assorted berries (such as strawberries, blueberries, raspberries, or blackberries), washed and sliced if needed

Instructions:

1. Place the milk, chia seeds, vanilla essence, maple syrup (or honey, if using), in a jar or mixing bowl. Mix well to blend.
2. To allow the chia seeds to thicken and absorb the liquid, cover the dish or jar and refrigerate the chia seed

mixture for at least 4 hours, but ideally overnight. To avoid clumping, stir or shake occasionally while the food is refrigerated.

3. Give the chia seed pudding one last stir when it has thickened to the consistency you like.
4. Spoon the chia seed pudding into separate dishes or serving cups for dishing.
5. Place a variety of fruit on top of the chia seed pudding.
6. For added sweetness, you may want to sprinkle a bit more honey or maple syrup over the berries.
7. Serve right away and savor your delectable Chia Seed Pudding with Berries as a wholesome choice for dessert, breakfast, or a snack.

12. Energy Balls Made with Dates, Nuts, and Coconut

Ingredients:

- 1 cup Medjool dates, pitted
- 1 cup nuts of your choice (such as almonds, cashews, walnuts, or a mix), unsalted
- 1/4 cup shredded coconut (plus extra for rolling, if desired)

- 1 tablespoon chia seeds or flaxseeds (optional, for extra nutrition)
- 1 tablespoon cocoa powder or cacao powder (optional, for chocolate flavor)
- 1/2 teaspoon vanilla extract
- Pinch of salt (optional)

Instructions:

1. Transfer the pitted dates to a food processor and pulse until they create a sticky paste and are finely chopped.
2. Transfer the nuts, shredded coconut, vanilla essence, chia or flax seeds, cocoa powder, or cacao powder, and a little teaspoon of salt (if using) to the food processor.
3. Pulse the ingredients to create a sticky dough by coarsely chopping the nuts and mixing them in thoroughly with the dates.
4. You can add a small amount of water, one tablespoon at a time, if the mixture looks too dry, until it comes together easily when pushed between your fingers.
5. Using your hands, roll tablespoon-sized parts of the mixture into balls.
6. You can choose to cover the outside of the energy balls by rolling them in crushed coconut.
7. To solidify, place the energy balls on a baking sheet covered with parchment paper and chill for a minimum of half an hour.

8. The energy balls are ready to eat after they've chilled. Any leftovers can be kept in the fridge for up to a week if they are kept in an airtight container.

13. Frozen Yogurt Bark with Granola and Fruit

Ingredients:

- 2 cups Greek yogurt (plain or flavored)
- 1/4 cup honey or maple syrup
- 1 teaspoon vanilla extract
- 1/2 cup granola
- Assorted fresh fruit (such as berries, sliced bananas, kiwi, mango, etc.), washed and chopped if needed

Instructions:

1. Place the Greek yogurt, vanilla extract, and honey (or maple syrup) in a mixing dish. Mix well until fully incorporated.
2. Use silicone baking mats or parchment paper to line a baking pan.
3. Transfer the Greek yogurt mixture to the baking sheet that has been preheated, and level it out into a layer that is between 1/4 and 1/2 inch thick.

4. Evenly scatter the granola on top of the layer of Greek yogurt.
5. Scatter the mixed fresh fruit on top of the granola and gently push it into the yogurt mixture.
6. Put the baking sheet in the freezer and freeze the yogurt bark until it solidifies, which should take at least two to three hours.
7. After the yogurt bark has frozen, take it out of the freezer and use a knife or your hands to break it into pieces.
8. Serve right away as a wholesome and cooling snack or dessert choice.

14. Popcorn Sprinkled with Nutritional Yeast

Ingredients:

- 1/4 cup popcorn kernels
- 2 tablespoons nutritional yeast
- 1-2 tablespoons melted butter or olive oil
- Salt to taste

Instructions:

1. Follow the manufacturer's directions for popping the popcorn kernels using an air popper, stovetop popper, or microwave. Ensure that the kernels pop all the way.
2. Pour the popcorn that has been popped into a large mixing dish.
3. Pour some melted butter or olive oil on the popcorn and gently toss to coat all over.
4. After properly coating the popcorn with a second toss, sprinkle it with nutritional yeast.
5. Season to taste with salt and toss again to evenly spread the seasoning.
6. Serve right away and savor your tasty popcorn that has been sprinkled with nutritional yeast as a nutritious and delectable snack.

15. Dark Chocolate Squares with a Handful of Nuts

Ingredients:

- Dark chocolate bars or squares (at least 70% cocoa)
- Assorted nuts (such as almonds, walnuts, pecans, hazelnuts, etc.)

Instructions:

1. Use silicone baking mats or parchment paper to line a baking pan.
2. If the dark chocolate bars aren't already divided into separate portions, break them into squares or pieces.
3. Arrange the squares of dark chocolate, allowing space between them, on the baking sheet that has been prepared.
4. If preferred, coarsely cut the various nuts into smaller bits in a small dish.
5. Gently press a handful of chopped nuts into the chocolate on top of each square of dark chocolate.
6. Refrigerate the baking sheet for ten to fifteen minutes, or until the nuts and chocolate are set.
7. Take the dark chocolate pieces out of the fridge after the chocolate has solidified.
8. As a rich and filling alternative for a snack or dessert, serve your delectable Dark Chocolate Squares with a Handful of Nuts right away.

CHAPTER EIGHT

TASTY AND NUTRITIOUS SMOOTHIE RECIPES TO SOOTHE YOUR CRAVINGS

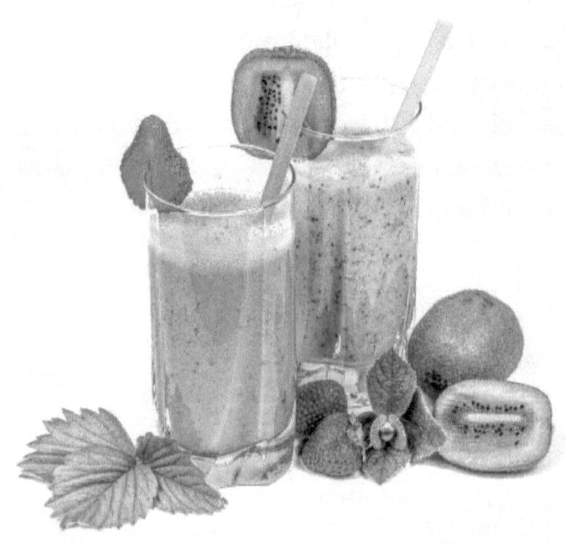

1. Berry Blast Smoothie

Ingredients:

- 1 cup mixed berries (such as strawberries, blueberries, raspberries, and blackberries), fresh or frozen
- 1/2 banana, fresh or frozen (for added sweetness and creaminess)
- 1/2 cup plain Greek yogurt (or dairy-free yogurt for a vegan option)
- 1/2 cup unsweetened almond milk (or any milk of your choice)
- 1 tablespoon honey or maple syrup (optional, for added sweetness)
- 1/2 teaspoon vanilla extract (optional, for extra flavor)
- Ice cubes (if using fresh berries)

Instructions:

1. Fill the blender with all the ingredients.
2. Process on high speed until smooth and creamy; adjust consistency with additional almond milk if needed.
3. If preferred, add extra honey or maple syrup to taste and adjust sweetness.
4. Transfer the smoothie into cups and start serving right away.

2. Green Goddess Smoothie

Ingredients:

- 1 cup fresh spinach leaves
- 1/2 ripe banana
- 1/2 cup chopped cucumber
- 1/2 cup chopped pineapple (fresh or frozen)
- 1/2 avocado
- 1 tablespoon fresh lemon juice
- 1/2 cup unsweetened almond milk (or any milk of your choice)
- Ice cubes (optional)

Instructions:

1. In a blender, combine all the ingredients.
2. Blend on high speed until smooth and creamy, adding extra almond milk as needed to get the consistency you want.
3. If desired, add extra lemon juice after tasting to modify the flavor.
4. Add a few ice cubes and end until smooth again if you'd like your smoothie to be cooler.
5. Fill glasses with the smoothie and serve right away.

3. Tropical Paradise Smoothie

Ingredients:

- 1 cup frozen pineapple chunks
- 1/2 cup frozen mango chunks
- 1/2 banana
- 1/2 cup coconut milk (or any milk of your choice)
- 1/2 cup Greek yogurt (plain or vanilla)
- 1 tablespoon honey or maple syrup (optional, for added sweetness)
- Juice of 1/2 lime (optional, for extra tanginess)
- Ice cubes (optional, for a colder smoothie)

Instructions:

1. Fill the blender with all the ingredients.
2. Process on high speed until smooth and creamy; adjust consistency with additional coconut milk if needed.
3. If preferred, add extra honey or maple syrup to taste and adjust sweetness.
4. Add the juice of half a lime for an additional flavor boost, and mix until combined.
5. You may add a few ice cubes and blend the smoothie again until it's smooth if you'd like it cooler.

6. Transfer the smoothie into glasses, and if preferred, top with more pineapple chunks or shredded coconut.
7. Pour over your Tropical Paradise Smoothie right away and savor this cool, tropical delight!

4. Peanut Butter Banana Smoothie

Ingredients:

- 1 ripe banana
- 1 tablespoon peanut butter (creamy or crunchy)
- 1/2 cup Greek yogurt (plain or vanilla)
- 1/2 cup milk (dairy or plant-based)
- 1 tablespoon honey or maple syrup (optional, for added sweetness)
- Ice cubes (optional, for a colder smoothie)

Instructions:

1. After peeling, chop the banana into large pieces.
2. Put the banana chunks, Greek yogurt, peanut butter, milk, honey, or maple syrup (if using) in a blender.
3. Add a couple ice cubes to the blender if you'd like your smoothie cooler.

4. Blend on high speed until smooth and creamy, stopping the blender as necessary to scrape down the sides.
5. After tasting the smoothie, taste it and, if needed, add additional honey or maple syrup to regulate the sweetness.
6. Immediately serve the smoothie by pouring it into glasses.

5. Chocolate Avocado Smoothie

Ingredients:

- 1 ripe avocado
- 1 ripe banana
- 2 tablespoons cocoa powder (unsweetened)
- 1 tablespoon honey or maple syrup (optional, for added sweetness)
- 1 cup milk of your choice (dairy or plant-based)
- Ice cubes (optional, for a colder smoothie)
- Optional toppings: shaved dark chocolate, sliced banana, or a sprinkle of cocoa powder

Instructions:

1. Halve the avocado, remove the pit, and extract the flesh with a spoon.

2. After peeling, chop the banana into small pieces.
3. Put the avocado, banana, milk, cocoa powder, honey (if using), and maple syrup in a blender.
4. Add a couple ice cubes to the blender if you'd like your smoothie cooler.
5. Blend on high speed until smooth and creamy, stopping the blender as necessary to scrape down the sides.
6. After tasting the smoothie, taste it and, if needed, add more honey or maple syrup to balance sweetness.
7. Immediately serve the smoothie by pouring it into glasses.
8. For an extra-indulgent touch, you might choose to top with sliced banana, shaved dark chocolate, or cocoa powder.

6. Mango Pineapple Smoothie

Ingredients:

- 1 cup frozen mango chunks
- 1 cup frozen pineapple chunks
- 1/2 banana (fresh or frozen, for creaminess)
- 1/2 cup Greek yogurt (plain or vanilla)
- 1/2 cup coconut water or water
- Optional: honey or maple syrup, to taste (if additional sweetness is desired)

- **Optional:** ice cubes, for a colder smoothie

Instructions:

1. In a blender, combine the frozen mango and pineapple pieces, banana, Greek yogurt, and coconut water (or water).
2. You may also add a few ice cubes to the blender if you'd want your smoothie to be cooler.
3. Blend at a high speed until the mixture is smooth and creamy and all the ingredients are properly blended. To make sure all the ingredients are incorporated equally, pause the blender if necessary and use a spatula to scrape along the edges.
4. If you want a sweeter flavor, taste the smoothie and add honey or maple syrup.
5. Transfer the smoothie into glasses after the right sweetness and smoothness have been reached.
6. Pour and enjoy your cool mango-pineapple smoothie right now!

7. Strawberry Spinach Smoothie

Ingredients:

- 1 cup fresh spinach leaves

- 1 cup frozen strawberries
- 1/2 banana (fresh or frozen, for creaminess)
- 1/2 cup Greek yogurt (plain or vanilla)
- 1/2 cup milk of your choice (dairy or plant-based)
- Optional: honey or maple syrup, to taste (if additional sweetness is desired)
- **Optional:** ice cubes, for a colder smoothie

Instructions:

1. Fill the blender with the frozen strawberries, banana, Greek yogurt, fresh spinach leaves, and milk.
2. You may also add a few ice cubes to the blender if you'd want your smoothie to be cooler.
3. Blend at a high speed until the mixture is smooth and creamy and all the ingredients are properly blended. To make sure all the ingredients are incorporated equally, pause the blender and use a spatula to scrape along the edges.
4. If you want a sweeter flavor, taste the smoothie and add honey or maple syrup.
5. Transfer the smoothie into glasses after the right sweetness and smoothness have been reached.
6. Pour and savor your wholesome Strawberry Spinach Smoothie right now!

8. Blueberry Almond Smoothie

Ingredients:

- 1 cup frozen blueberries
- 1/2 banana (fresh or frozen, for creaminess)
- 1 tablespoon almond butter
- 1/2 cup Greek yogurt (plain or vanilla)
- 1/2 cup almond milk (or any milk of your choice)
- Optional: honey or maple syrup, to taste (if additional sweetness is desired)
- **Optional:** ice cubes, for a colder smoothie

Instructions:

1. Fill a blender with the frozen blueberries, banana, Greek yogurt, almond butter, and almond milk.
2. You may also add a few ice cubes to the blender if you'd want your smoothie to be cooler.
3. Blend at a high speed until the mixture is smooth and creamy and all the ingredients are properly blended. To make sure all the ingredients are incorporated equally, pause the blender and use a spatula to scrape along the edges.
4. If you want a sweeter flavor, taste the smoothie and add honey or maple syrup.
5. Transfer the smoothie into glasses after the right sweetness and smoothness have been reached.

6. Pour and savor your delectable Blueberry Almond Smoothie right away!

9. Peachy Keen Smoothie

Ingredients:

- 1 cup frozen peach slices
- 1/2 banana (fresh or frozen, for creaminess)
- 1/2 cup Greek yogurt (plain or vanilla)
- 1/2 cup orange juice (or any juice of your choice)
- 1/4 teaspoon vanilla extract
- **Optional:** honey or maple syrup, to taste (if additional sweetness is desired)
- **Optional:** ice cubes, for a colder smoothie

Instructions:

1. In a blender, combine the banana, Greek yogurt, orange juice, frozen peach segments, and vanilla essence.
2. You may also add a few ice cubes to the blender if you'd want your smoothie to be cooler.
3. Blend at a high speed until the mixture is smooth and creamy and all the ingredients are properly blended. To make sure all the ingredients are incorporated equally,

pause the blender and use a spatula to scrape along the edges.

4. If you want a sweeter flavor, taste the smoothie and add honey or maple syrup.

5. Transfer the smoothie into glasses after the right sweetness and smoothness have been reached.

6. Pour into glasses right away and savor your Peachy Keen Smoothie!

10. Creamy Coconut Smoothie

Ingredients:

- 1/2 cup canned coconut milk (full-fat for creaminess)
- 1/2 cup coconut water (or regular water)
- 1/2 cup Greek yogurt (plain or vanilla)
- 1/2 cup frozen pineapple chunks
- 1/2 banana (fresh or frozen, for sweetness and creaminess)
- **Optional:** honey or maple syrup, to taste (if additional sweetness is desired)
- **Optional:** shredded coconut or coconut flakes, for garnish

Instructions:

1. Put the Greek yogurt, frozen pineapple pieces, banana, canned coconut milk, and coconut water in a blender.
2. Blend at a high speed until the mixture is smooth and creamy and all the ingredients are well blended. To make sure all the ingredients are incorporated equally, pause the blender if necessary and use a spatula to scrape along the edges.
3. If you want a sweeter flavor, taste the smoothie and add honey or maple syrup.
4. Transfer the smoothie into glasses after the right sweetness and smoothness have been reached.
5. For more coconut taste and texture, you can choose to add shredded coconut or coconut flakes to the smoothie as a garnish.
6. Present your velvety Coconut Smoothie right away and savor it!

11. Kiwi Kale Smoothie

Ingredients:

- 1 kiwi, peeled and sliced
- 1 cup fresh kale leaves, stems removed
- 1/2 banana (fresh or frozen, for sweetness and creaminess)
- 1/2 cup Greek yogurt (plain or vanilla)
- 1/2 cup coconut water (or water)

- **Optional:** honey or maple syrup, to taste (if additional sweetness is desired)
- **Optional:** ice cubes, for a colder smoothie

Instructions:

1. In a blender, combine the banana, Greek yogurt, coconut water, kiwi slices, and fresh kale leaves.
2. You may also add a few ice cubes to the blender if you'd want your smoothie to be cooler.
3. Blend at a high speed until the mixture is smooth and creamy and all the ingredients are properly blended. To make sure all the ingredients are incorporated equally, pause the blender and use a spatula to scrape along the edges.
4. If you want a sweeter flavor, taste the smoothie and add honey or maple syrup.
5. Transfer the smoothie into glasses after the right sweetness and smoothness have been reached.
6. Pour and savor your wholesome Kiwi Kale Smoothie right away!

12. Orange Creamsicle Smoothie

Ingredients:

- 1 large orange, peeled and segmented

- 1/2 banana (fresh or frozen, for creaminess)
- 1/2 cup Greek yogurt (plain or vanilla)
- 1/2 cup milk (dairy or plant-based)
- 1/2 teaspoon vanilla extract
- **Optional:** honey or maple syrup, to taste (if additional sweetness is desired)
- **Optional:** ice cubes, for a colder smoothie

Instructions:

1. Fill a blender with the orange segments, banana, Greek yogurt, milk, and essence from vanilla.
2. You may also add a few ice cubes to the blender if you'd want your smoothie to be cooler.
3. Blend at a high speed until the mixture is smooth and creamy and all the ingredients are properly blended. To make sure all the ingredients are incorporated equally, pause the blender and use a spatula to scrape along the edges.
4. If you want a sweeter flavor, taste the smoothie and add honey or maple syrup.
5. Transfer the smoothie into glasses after the right sweetness and smoothness have been reached.
6. Pour and savor your Orange Creamsicle Smoothie right away!

CONCLUSION

As our adventure through the **Stage 4 Breast Cancer Diet Cookbook** draws to a close, I hope that these pages have empowered, soothed, and inspired you. Living with stage 4 breast cancer comes with obstacles, but you can manage your health and well-being via diet if you have the correct information and resources.

We've looked at a range of delectable and healthy meals in this cookbook that are especially meant to help people with stage 4 breast cancer. Every meal, from colorful smoothies overflowing with antioxidants to substantial salads loaded with fiber and protein, has been thoughtfully prepared to nurture the body and the soul.

Beyond only the dishes, though, this cookbook seeks to enlighten and educate. We have explored the scientific basis of how specific diets and nutrients might affect the course of cancer and the effectiveness of treatment. Knowing how diet plays a part in managing cancer will

help you make decisions that will improve your general health and quality of life.
While nutrition is an important component of cancer therapy, it is vital to keep in mind that it is only one part of the picture. In addition to eating healthfully, maintaining a holistic approach to well-being is crucial. This entails maintaining an active lifestyle, controlling stress, obtaining adequate sleep, and asking for help from loved ones, healthcare providers, and neighborhood services.

Recognize that you are not alone as you manage the challenges of living with stage 4 breast cancer. This cookbook is your travel companion, providing you with helpful advice, delectable recipes, and inspirational sayings to help you along the journey. Whether you're preparing food for a loved one, yourself, or a caregiver, I hope these recipes will make you happy and healthy.

To conclude, I would like to sincerely thank everyone who helped to make this cookbook possible. This book is a monument to the strength of community and cooperation, from the researchers and medical experts who work persistently to expand our knowledge of cancer nutrition to the home cooks and chefs who inspire us with their culinary creations.

My thoughts are with all the people and families who have been impacted by stage 4 breast cancer. In the kitchen and elsewhere, may you discover fortitude, resiliency, and optimism. Recall that food can bring people together, heal, and soothe. Let us celebrate life and show perseverance in the face of hardship by appreciating each meal.

I appreciate you traveling with me on this trip. I hope your kitchen is constantly stocked with good food, love, and laughter.

Sincerely,

[Kathleen Scribner]

www.ingramcontent.com/pod-product-compliance
Lightning Source LLC
Chambersburg PA
CBHW051259250726
48656CB00004B/1375

* 9 7 9 8 3 2 2 4 7 8 2 2 5 *